"You're on the Air with Dr. Fratellone"

"You're on the Air with Dr. Fratellone"

◆

Answers to Questions Most Frequently Asked About Supplements and Herbs for the Heart

"Dr. Fratellone may well be one of the most outstanding complementary cardiologists in the nation."
—Robert C. Atkins, MD

*Patrick M. Fratellone, MD and
Barbara Mendez, RPh*

iUniverse, Inc.
New York Lincoln Shanghai

"You're on the Air with Dr. Fratellone"
Answers to Questions Most Frequently Asked About Supplements and Herbs for the Heart

Copyright © 2005 by RPG Associates, Inc.

All rights reserved. No part of this book may be used or reproduced by any means, graphic, electronic, or mechanical, including photocopying, recording, taping or by any information storage retrieval system without the written permission of the publisher except in the case of brief quotations embodied in critical articles and reviews.

iUniverse books may be ordered through booksellers or by contacting:

iUniverse
2021 Pine Lake Road, Suite 100
Lincoln, NE 68512
www.iuniverse.com
1-800-Authors (1-800-288-4677)

This book is dedicated to providing the public and health professionals with scientific information related to vitamins and heart disease. It is not intended as medical advice. Our purpose for this publication is solely informational and educational. Please consult a physician or other health professional should the need for one be warranted.

The mention of companies or product trade names does not constitute an endorsement of them by the authors or RPG Associates Inc. and is done solely for the purpose of providing relevant information to our readers.

ISBN: 0-595-32647-1 (pbk)
ISBN: 0-595-66660-4 (cloth)

Printed in the United States of America

This book is dedicated to all my radio listeners. Your questions have given life to the premise of this project: through your questions, you help me to educate others.

My life would not be complete if not for the unconventional love, compassion, and trust of my two children, Alyssa and Gregory, and my beloved father, Pat, Sr.

And finally, looking down upon me, one soul—my mother.

I could not have done this without each of you.

My sincere thanks are extended to my wonderful staff at The Fratellone Group for their day-to-day support and also to Greg Schraer, Arthur Stein, Tina Discepola, Fred and Nancy Byrd, and Rick Byrd.

Contents

Foreword xi

Introduction xiii

Section I. Vita-Nutrients for the Heart 1
    Vita-Nutrients for the Heart 2
    Nutritional Supplements 3
    Treating Conditions with Nutritional Supplements 16
    Supplements for Male and Female Health 28

Section II. Herbs for the Heart 35
    Herbs for the Heart 36

Section III. Addressing Specific Cardiac Conditions with
    Integrative Approaches 43
    Cardiovascular Disease and the Use of Supplements and Herbs ... 44
    Coronary Artery Disease 44
    Hyperlipidemia 62
    Arrhythmias 69
    Valvular Heart Disease, Cardiomyopathy, and Congestive Heart
        Failure 78
    Hypertension 86

Conclusion 93

Glossary 95

Bibliography 101

About the Fratellone Group for Integrative Cardiology and
    Medicine 103

About Longevity Nutritional Products and Services 105

Index 107

THE ATKINS CENTER FOR
COMPLEMENTARY MEDICINE

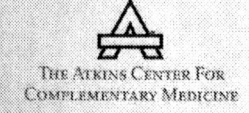

June 4, 2002

To Whom It May Concern:

Re: Dr. Patrick Fratellone

For three years, Dr. Fratellone was the chief cardiologist at the Atkins Center for Complementary Medicine. He was quickly given the second post as medical director, as well.

Dr. Fratellone may well be one of the most outstanding complementary cardiologists in the nation. He focuses on finding the cause of heart disease, looking for infection, elevated triglycerides, homocysteine, lipoprotein(a), fibrinogen, as well as the standard concern over cholesterol. He offers a different solution for each condition.

Dr. Fratellone is experienced with EECP, elimination of infections, use of vitanutrients capable of reversing heart disease, in addition to the standard therapies used in cardiology.

His work ethic is excellent; he is devoted to seeing long lists of patients. He also is very good at speaking on these subjects to lay people as well as professionals.

Sincerely,

Robert C. Atkins, M.D.

Foreword

If you happen to be one of the thousands of listeners or callers who have listened to my weekly radio programs in the New York City area, then you have no doubt heard me say, "You're on the air with Dr. Fratellone."

It has long been my desire to educate my radio listeners and now you, the reader, on safe alternatives to conventional medicine. This desire has prompted me to publish this book, which is based on questions frequently asked by patients and other interested persons who called into my radio show, *House Calls with Dr. Fratellone*, on WWRL, 1600 kHz AM, in the New York City area (via the Internet, www.wwrl1600.com). This book is intended as an introductory guide to a healthy heart. No part of this book represents a treatment plan; the book is merely a guide to some of the options available to those who are seeking them.

For years, I have used radio as an extension of my office practice. I consider radio and television as valuable tools for reaching individuals outside my practice, such as people who are ill and homebound, people who have questions that need answering but who feel uncomfortable asking their own physicians, and people who are interested in more than what conventional medicine can provide. In addition, I receive thousands of questions via our website, www.thefratellonegroup.com, relating to heart disease.

As an *integrative cardiologist* and an *internist*, I practice medicine by incorporating the best of conventional medicine with alternative treatments. More and more people are interested in how to treat and combat disease through the use of vitamins, minerals, and other supplements.

In our practice, co-author Barbara Mendez and I each meet with our patients to ensure that they receive professional, one-on-one answers to all of their medical questions. Nevertheless, I trust that you will find the answers to many of your questions by reading this book. So sit back, relax, and pretend that you've tuned in to hear, *"You're on the air with Dr. Fratellone."*

Introduction

As a group, cardiovascular disease causes more deaths than any other disease known to humanity; unfortunately, more than 60 million Americans suffer from some form of this disease of the blood vessels that serve the heart (referred to as the *cardiovascular* system), including high blood pressure, heart-rhythm problems, coronary artery disease, and congestive heart failure. Coronary artery disease alone accounts for over half a million deaths annually.

Over the last several decades, advancements in technology have led to improvements in clinical care. But despite such medical progress and greater public awareness, coronary artery disease is still a leading health risk, one that makes those who suffer from it vulnerable to such debilitating consequences as angina (chest pain) and stroke. Sadly, once cardiovascular disease develops, it cannot be cured, only managed. Thus, the ultimate key to survival is prevention. In particular, our emphasis today needs to be placed on the control of two epidemics: diabetes and obesity, both factors that contribute to heart disease.

Millions of dollars are spent each year on advertising that focuses on the known risk factors for heart disease, such as hypertension (high blood pressure) and elevated total cholesterol, yet many other cardiovascular risk factors go largely ignored. As a culture, we seem to be hooked on treating cholesterol levels and especially "bad" cholesterol (low-density lipoproteins [LDL]) with ever-new-and-evolving drugs that banish bad cholesterol, and sometimes doing so without enough regard to potentially dangerous side effects. Many studies suggest that the best ways of preventing cardiovascular disease are by modifying the behaviors that predispose us to, or make us more susceptible to, risk—such as quitting smoking, increasing exercise, and modifying our diets. Yet we are still, as a culture, fixated on obtaining easy solutions, which require little or no participation on our part. Not enough attention is focused on behavior modifications, while drug companies become richer and we as a nation become fatter and sicker.

In addition, other cardiac risk factors, which I term Longevity Risk Factors™, are largely ignored. These risk factors—which are each individually defined in the Glossary at the back of this book and are discussed throughout—include homocysteine, lipoprotein(a), fibrinogen, and high-sensitivity C-reactive protein. These factors are as detrimental to cardiac health as elevated cholesterol, and, in some cases, more so. These largely unacknowledged risk factors can create disease in the circulatory system and heart muscle with as much destructive capability as hypertension or high cholesterol. Ironically, advertisers depict cholesterol as a deadly poison that should be reduced to absurdly low levels, yet a *healthy cholesterol level* is vital to all human cells. Recent research studies, funded by large drug corporations, suggest that cholesterol levels should be maintained at ridiculously low levels through the use of one or another *statin* drug, while ignoring the implications of such recommendations, which include impotence and exacerbated stress levels. In my own practice (and in many physicians' offices), muscle aches and weakness occur in approximately 30% of patients who take statins. In 2001, a consumer group called Public Citizen discovered that statin drugs were linked to 72 fatal and 772 nonfatal cases of rhabdomyolysis (muscle tissue breakdown) between October 1997 and December 2000. Also of note is that in 2001, the statin Baycol® (cerivastatin) was removed from the market after it was linked to 31 deaths.

Mainstream solutions to heart disease focus on invasive procedures, including angioplasty, the use of stents, and coronary bypass grafting, after conventional prescribed medications have failed to yield results. Unfortunately, these procedures may provide only temporary solutions for symptomatic relief, and may lead to complications. In many cases, invasive procedures are unnecessary and produce no great benefits. To be clear, I am not opposed to invasive procedures or coronary artery surgery, but I believe that they should be used as an absolute last resort, after all other interventions have failed. For example, before considering such invasive procedures, I discuss alternative options with my patients such as the importance of a healthy, balanced diet and the need for exercise. Additionally, I employ an array of alternative and integrative options, such as acupuncture, EECP® (enhanced external counterpulsation), chelation therapy, and Plaquex®. These therapies are safer, simpler, and far less expensive than invasive options, and most, if not all, can be done in the doctor's office, eliminating the need for a hospital stay.

As an integrative physician, I begin by conducting a complete history and physical examination of each patient, taking into account dietary and nutritional history as well as exercise and lifestyle considerations. The use of vitamins, minerals, herbs, and other supplements is addressed and reviewed for efficacy and necessity. The management and treatment of heart disease begins here. After reviewing the results of tests on the patient's blood chemistry as well as other test results, a treatment plan is recommended that includes dietary changes, if necessary; the addition or elimination of supplements and medications, as needed; and the adoption of other integrative practices. Follow-ups are conducted in a timely fashion as we keep a sharp eye on patient progress and improvement.

Remember that this book is meant to be used as a guide to having a healthy heart and should be considered as such. It does not contain treatment plans, but it does offer you some alternatives.

Section I.

Vita-Nutrients for the Heart

Vita-Nutrients for the Heart

It is estimated that more than 60% of all health care consumers take some form of a vitamin, alone or in combination with their conventional medications. Because of this prevalence, we as physicians need to be better informed about supplement interactions with conventional medications as well as with other supplements. After much reading; by attending symposiums and courses; through learning from my previous mentor, the late Robert C. Atkins, MD; and through my current involvement with the Associative Fellowship of Integrative Medicine with Andrew Weil, MD; I am comfortable and confident in discussing supplements.

Of great concern is the fact that patients who use alternative therapies seldom discuss or mention their use with their conventional health care practitioners. As is mentioned throughout this book, it is important for all patients to discuss with their doctors the use of over-the-counter supplements. Likewise, it is important for physicians to broaden their scope to include alternative therapies.

This book contains answers to your commonly asked questions regarding the safe use of herbs, vitamins, minerals, and similar substances sometimes collectively referred to as *vita-nutrients*. The book is intended to educate you, the consumer, as well as health care practitioners.

Nutritional Supplements

You're on the Air...
Q. Where can I find a comprehensive list of uses for vitamins?

A. One of the best guides for the use of supplements is the book *Prescription for Nutritional Healing,* third edition, by Phyllis A. and James F. Balch. The text alphabetically classifies diseases and provides a list of supplements that would benefit each condition. It also has a section devoted to each category of supplement (vitamins, minerals, amino acids, herbs, etc.). It is very thorough and comprehensive. Another choice would be *The Best Supplement Guide for Your Health,* by Don Goldberg, RPh and Arnold Gitomer, RPh, which is a complete list of all the nutritional supplements available, their uses, and the best brand to buy for each nutrient. Written by two pharmacists that own the largest holistic pharmacy in the United States, Willner Chemists, this book is very practical and can guide the consumer through the myriad of options available.

Q. I am a vegetarian. Can you recommend vegetarian sources for vitamins and supplements? Vegetarians do not want to ingest gelatin capsules, and finding a substitute is most difficult. Do you have any suggestions?

A. Solgar® is a supplement manufacturer that provides many of their products in vegetable capsules, which would be appropriate. By contrast, tablets are often suitable for vegetarians, but read the list of ingredients to make sure that they are free of dairy, starch, corn, and sugar fillers and binders.

Q. What is the difference between vitamins and supplements?

A. Technically speaking, supplements are intended to add nutrients that may be lacking in the diet, whereas vitamins are ingested to support various processes in the body. These terms are often used interchangeably. Frequently, diet alone is not sufficient in meeting the needs of the human body. Individuals who skip meals, eat junk food, or rely on coffee and soda to get through the day with little regard for fruits and vegetables and other whole foods will probably benefit from the use of vitamins and other supplements to compensate for what is lacking in their diets.

Q. Are liquid vitamins better than pills and gels?

A. Liquid vitamins tend to have a faster absorption rate than pills because the vitamins are already dissolved and don't need to be broken down by stomach acids, as do pills. However, liquid supplements are not the most economical way to take nutrients. Because most people can swallow pills and tend to prefer that to having to taste a liquid they may not like, liquids are not widely distributed, thereby making them more expensive.

Gels or creams applied to the body are good ways to transport certain medications, such as hormones for replacement therapy in women during and after menopause, but in general they are not used for transporting vitamins and minerals.

If you are concerned about absorption, take capsules. Capsules are easier to digest than tablets. If you are buying a fat-soluble supplement, such as vitamins A or E or coenzyme Q_{10} (CoQ_{10}), a gel cap would increase the absorption by as much as 30% compared with dry powder capsules.

Q. What does the % Daily Value on Nutrition Facts panels mean? How do I know if I am getting too much or not enough?

A. Such labels usually reflect what is absolutely necessary for the human body to consume in order to prevent disease or death. However, the percentages are not an indication of what is optimal to promote health, vitality, and longevity. For instance, do not be alarmed when a supplement states that it contains 200% of the daily requirement. This only means that, for that particular nutrient, small doses are needed to prevent illness. Usually, supplements are made with therapeutic doses in mind—meaning the dose needed to exert a positive influence in the body. For example, it is only necessary to consume 1 mg (milligram) of vitamin B_1 per day to meet the requirement necessary as estimated by the some U.S. governmental units. In adult multivitamin formulas, B_1 is often included in doses that range from 15 to 100 mg. Such doses are perfectly safe as long as you or your health care practitioner sets up your regimen with the appropriate proportions of other B vitamins, which are best taken as a group.

Q. When you go to the drug store to select vitamins, how do you know which ones are most effective?

A. It's best to buy your supplements from a vitamin store or pharmacy whose staff members are knowledgeable about the various manufacturers and can guide you through the process. There is no real way to determine quality, but it would be wise to purchase vitamins that are hypoallergenic. Hypoallergenic supplements are free of corn, wheat, dairy, sugar, and starch. There is also a website, consumerlab.com, that evaluates supplement product lines, lists the highest quality nutrients available, and makes note of those brands that fall under par.

Q. Are there any health risks from taking any vitamins and minerals?

A. If taken wisely, and under the supervision of a licensed and knowledgeable practitioner, vitamins and minerals are very safe to take and it is rare that a consumer will encounter a problem. However, caution should be used when taking the fat-soluble vitamins, such as A, E, and D, and the substance CoQ_{10}. Because these nutrients are stored in fat, they can accumulate when taken in large doses and cause toxicity in the liver. To prevent vitamin toxicity, take your vitamins only as recommended or prescribed.

Caution should also be used when combining vitamins, minerals, and especially herbs with prescribed medications, as there could be an interaction. For example, a patient on Coumadin®, a common blood thinner, should take vitamin E only under the supervision of a doctor. There are other such interactions, so before beginning a supplement regimen, be sure to consult a knowledgeable practitioner who can help you combine the two modes of treatment.

Q. Why do we need vitamins? Are they not already supplied in the foods we eat?

A. If you are inclined toward a whole foods diet, then yes, you should be receiving the nutrients you need to survive from your food. By "whole foods diet," I mean plenty of vegetables, fruits, beans, nuts, and seeds. A whole foods diet can include meats—fish, chicken, and occasionally red meat—preferable from animals raised on organically grown feed products. If you can eat this way all the time, with fresh food, not frozen, canned, or overly processed, then you are probably doing okay. However, how many people do you know who eat this way consistently? Not many, I suspect. Most people eat too many refined carbohydrates, like bread, bagels, and pasta, not to mention the sugars found in candy, cakes, cookies, and muffins. If you add coffee consumption to this, which is a diuretic and enhances the loss of vital minerals from the body, and then throw in the frozen dinner or a take-out meal, what you are actually consuming is a plateful of *macronutrients* (fat, protein, and carbohydrates). The subtle *micronutrients* get washed away in the preparation, canning, and freezing, and cooking of these products. So we're eating, as a nation, more than ever before: we are malnourished, yet obese. This is a direct correlation to the fact that what we are eating is depleted of life-sustaining vitamins and minerals. This is why almost all people can benefit from the use of supplements.

Q. What is the difference between a water-soluble vitamin and a fat-soluble vitamin?

A. Water-soluble vitamins include vitamin C and the B vitamins, which consist of folic acid, B_{12}, B_6, pantothenic acid, thiamin, niacin, riboflavin, and biotin. Each of these vitamins must cross the intestinal wall and move into the bloodstream. Unlike the fat-soluble vitamins, water-soluble ones are not stored in the body and thus need to be replenished on a regular basis. And because the body does not hold onto the water-soluble vitamins, there are fewer potential side effects created by toxicity. Both the B vitamins and vitamin C are beneficial for cardiovascular disease, cancer prevention, macular degeneration (age-related loss of vision), and immune system dysfunction.

The fat-soluble vitamins include vitamin A, beta-carotene, CoQ_{10}, vitamin E, vitamin D, and vitamin K. Fat-soluble vitamins are stored in fat tissue and can accumulate if taken in excessive quantities. *Caution needs to be exercised when taking the fat-soluble supplements.*

Q. It is my understanding that certain vitamins and herbs are contraindicated when on certain medications. Is this true? Can you elaborate on this?

A. There are many vitamins and herbs that are contraindicated, meaning "should not be used," along with certain conventional medications. Since there is no regulatory body for the use of vitamins and herbs in this country, I caution all patients, including the reader of this book, to consult with a practitioner who can discuss the contraindications. In my field, cardiology, I am familiar with the interactions of many cardiac herbs and the use of the conventional medication classes, the beta-blockers and the calcium channel blockers.

For those individuals unable to see an integrative medical doctor, who is knowledgeable in treating patients with vitamins, herbs, and supplements, now in print are a *PDR® for Nutritional Supplements* and a *PDR® for Herbal Medicines, third edition,* that do indeed list the contraindications that supplements can have with a variety of conventional medications.

Q. How can we evaluate the recommendations of our physicians, if they are recommending vitamins and supplements, but clearly are not knowledgeable about them?

A. This poses an ethical question. As physicians, we do not gain our knowledge of supplements and nutrition from our courses in medical school. It takes a special dedication to the profession of healing. I have learned about supplements by readings and by attending courses, and am now enrolled in the Associative Fellowship of Integrative Medicine program with Andrew Weil, MD. My previous work experience with Robert C. Atkins, MD, set the groundwork on which I began to explore. Medicine has many facets. I continue to study the use of herbs, vitamins, and supplements in obtaining a healthy life. But I do agree with the Hippocratic oath in its admonition to harm no one, and I do believe the validity of Sir William Osler's quote that "medicine is taught at the bedside and not in the classroom." I have learned much from listening to my patients in regards to new herbs and vitamins that they read about. That being said, if you do not have confidence in what a medical practitioner is recommending to you, then seek out a second opinion with a knowledgeable professional. Do not follow medical advice blindly, especially if you do not trust that what is being suggested is in your best interest.

Q. Are there vitamins specifically for the heart?

A. I will list the top ten nutritional supplements for the heart here, and they will be discussed further in Section III of this book.

- Coenzyme Q_{10}
- The amino acid taurine
- The amino acid L-carnitine

- Magnesium
- The essential oils omega-3, omega-6, and docosahexaenoic acid (DHA)
- Vitamin E
- The herb hawthorn
- Vitamin C
- The B vitamins, especially folic acid and B_{12}
- Trace minerals (zinc and selenium)

Q. I recently started using coral calcium and, shortly thereafter, developed an arrhythmia. Is there any correlation, or is it just a coincidence?

A. Calcium is a vital nutrient not only for our bones, but also for the whole body. We do know that high-dose calcium can be used to help prevent osteoporosis. As a cardiologist, I am convinced that calcium can be used to lower blood pressure. I also combine calcium with magnesium to lower blood pressure, as it is more effective. Both these minerals can also help with arrhythmias. Nonetheless, it is possible that extra intake of either of these minerals can cause arrhythmias. You could develop an arrhythmia when your blood pressure becomes too low and this is a way your body compensates for the low blood pressure. The other cause is a possible allergy to calcium in its variety of forms. Because coral calcium comes from the coral reefs of Japan, there has been some evidence to suggest that this type of calcium may contain mercury. This is an important consideration because mercury toxicity can cause deleterious effects on the cardiovascular system, including arrhythmias and palpitations. My suggestion would be to discontinue the coral calcium and see whether the symptoms improve.

Q. How can I raise my calcium intake through food?

A. Although some dairy foods are appropriate sources of calcium, it is not recommended that you obtain all of your food sources of calcium through dairy. Eating too many dairy products can actually work against bone health because dairy is an acid-forming food that decreases the pH of the body. Technically speaking, when there is acidosis in the body, your bones begin to leach minerals in order to compensate, to alkalinize the body. This situation can worsen osteoporosis. However, sugar-free, low-fat yogurt does provide over 300 mg of calcium per cup and has the added benefit of providing acidophilus to the gut. Aside from yogurt and the occasional piece of cheese, you can also obtain calcium from dark-green leafy vegetables. Spinach, kale, bok choy, and broccoli also serve the purpose of alkalinizing the body, further contributing to the protection of bone density. Other sources include sardines (with bones that can be eaten), almonds, and calcium-enriched tofu.

Q. I have been told that I have too much iron in my blood. I am trying to maintain a low-fat, low-cholesterol, low-salt, and low-iron diet, which I find difficult to maintain. What would you recommend to help me maintain this type of diet?

A. You would benefit from a lean protein diet that includes chicken and fish with plenty of dark-green leafy vegetables. Avoid beef, liver, and most shellfish. Consuming larger quantities of dark-green leafy vegetables inhibits the absorption of iron, so it will help you in that regard as well as provide plenty of folic acid and calcium necessary for heart health. Drinking tea with or after meals also helps to inhibit iron absorption. For your particular condition, avoid taking extra vitamin C, as it enhances iron absorption. Vegetables such as broccoli, brussels sprouts, tomatoes, and peppers also enhance absorption and should be eaten in moderation. However, feel free to eat plenty of spinach and chard. Sweet potatoes are also iron inhibitors and a great alkalinizing food, so include half of one with lunch.

Q. I take 100 mg of CoQ$_{10}$ once a day and two 1,000-mg fish oil and two 1,000-mg flax oil capsules twice a day. Will taking these supplements help maintain a healthy heart?

A. Your regimen is adequate. However, a medical history and physical exam need to be performed to determine your regimen's adequacy in the light of your lifestyle, age, gender, and current use of conventional and alternative therapies. A blood analysis of other independent risk factors for heart disease needs to be obtained. These other risk factors are the levels of C-reactive protein (CRP), lipoprotein(a), fibrinogen, and homocysteine. I refer to these as the Longevity Risk Factors™. Certain vitamins can lower each of these risk factors. However, as a baseline, the regimen you are on is good. I recommend that you use flax seed oil instead of the capsules. The guideline for quantity of flax seed oil is one tablespoonful per one hundred pounds of body weight. You would need to take twelve capsules to get the equivalent of one tablespoonful of oil. All three of the nutrients you mentioned should be taken with food to enhance absorption.

Q. What are the most natural sources of omega-3?

A. The best sources of omega-3 fatty acids are salmon (wild Alaskan salmon), sardines, walnuts, and flax seeds. If taking flax, be sure to use the oil or ground seeds, because the whole seed is indigestible and thus beneficial only as a laxative. The dose of flax seed oil is one tablespoonful per hundred pounds of body weight. After taking the flax seed oil, with some food, have a cup of green tea for enhanced antioxidant activity and to promote heat throughout your body (thermogenesis). The dose of omega-3 fish oils will vary from person to person, but most will benefit from the addition of 1,000 mg of omega-3 fish oil (which amounts to one capsule daily) after food. Most people will require more for maintaining healthy fibrinogen levels, for improving circulation, and for the maintenance of healthy cholesterol levels.

Q. What is the best dosage for daily intake of vitamin C?

A. We now know that the single 8-oz. glass of orange juice is not adequate. There is a large volume of literature on the use of vitamin C. We must thank Nobel Prize winner Linus Pauling for his vision in the megadose theory of vitamin C. I cannot think of any disease in which vitamin C cannot exert some benefit. Whether it is cardiovascular disease, cancer, asthma, allergies, or infections, there is data to support its use. It is the most widely publicized *and criticized* vitamin. We do know that a deficiency leads to scurvy from historical data. Vitamin C should be given in divided doses starting with about 3 grams (3,000 mg) per day. I have found that you build up your vitamin C levels slowly increasing by 500 mg every other day. At higher doses of vitamin C, you will start to develop gastrointestinal side effects, such as diarrhea. This varies from patient to patient. Individuals who are deficient in vitamin C might reach intake levels of 9 grams before having the bowel intolerance. The individual then decreases their dosage by 500–1,000 mg, and that becomes their dosage. However, this changes in time as the body changes. A safe and effective dose is 1,000 to 3,000 mg, protecting your immune system and preventing free radical damage. The best form of vitamin C to take might be Ester C™, which is readily absorbed and does not upset the stomach. It also has a slight timed-release activity, which will keep it circulating in the body longer.

Q. While taking a multivitamin supplement, would it be okay to take extra vitamins A and D and also chromium?

A. Both vitamin A and D are fat-soluble vitamins and can accumulate in the body, thus possibly causing toxicity. Increased amounts in these vitamins should be monitored and used only for specific conditions.

An increase in vitamin A is often recommended for vision problems. Vitamin A in large doses has also been shown to be effective as an antibiotic, especially useful in bronchial infections and cystic acne. An increase in vitamin D is often recommended for bone problems, such as osteoporosis. It is reasonable to take 400 to 800 micrograms (mcg, or μg) per day of vitamin D for bone health because vitamin D helps the absorption of calcium and is a vital nutrient in the management of osteoporosis. Vitamin D in large doses has been shown to be effective in the treatment of psoriasis. High doses of vitamin D should not be taken alone and should be combined with calcium. *I would not recommend that anyone take high doses of any vitamin without the supervision of a knowledgeable and licensed practitioner.*

The mineral chromium is a pivotal vita-nutrient used to stabilize blood sugar and resensitize insulin-receptor sites, control cravings, and thereby lessening the desire to consume sugars. Chromium is also good to lower cholesterol levels and convert stored fat into energy and will enhance any eating plan geared toward targeting these areas. The recommended dose is 200 micrograms (mcg, or μg) one to three times per day on an empty stomach.

Q. What is the benefit of taking Coenzyme Q_{10}? I thought the body automatically produced CoQ_{10}.

A. The benefits of CoQ_{10} cannot be overstated! Also known as ubiquinone, CoQ_{10} helps to energize every cell in the body. It is great for enhancing performance and energy, weight loss, and promoting longevity. Taken in high doses, this nutrient also helps protect the heart from disease, protects the body from cancer, and can even help alleviate the symptoms of Parkinson's disease. It is a naturally occurring substance found in every living cell of the human body. It is found naturally in our foods, but with an average daily intake from food of no more than 10 mg. This amount is not substantial to achieve any beneficial results. Although present in some plant and animal cells, it can be found in higher concentrations in beef and pork heart, mackerel, broccoli, and spinach. It is best to take CoQ_{10} in a gel cap, as it is a fat-soluble nutrient and absorption is enhanced when taken in a gel cap form.

For those on cholesterol-lowering statin drugs, CoQ_{10} supplementation is essential because these drugs tend to lower CoQ_{10} in the body.

Q. What are the benefits of selenium?

A. This trace mineral has immunity-strengthening and cancer-preventive potential. It is a vital antioxidant. If an individual lacks selenium, they also lack an important enzyme called *glutathione peroxidase*. This mineral also helps our bodies fight viruses and bacteria. It has been used widely in the HIV population with changes in their immune function. Other conditions for which selenium has been used include inflammatory bowel disease, as in Crohn's and ulcerative colitis; osteoarthritis; thyroid disorders, metal toxicity, and pancreatitis. Selenium complements the absorption of vitamin E and these two nutrients should be taken together. Studies have shown that taking 200 to 300 micrograms (mcg, or µg) of selenium daily will help prevent breast and prostate cancers.

Q. Can I take too much vitamin E?

A. Vitamin E is a family of sixteen compounds. It is a fat-soluble vitamin and therefore can be stored in the fat, which can lead to toxicity in higher doses. Some reports suggest that a maximum dose can be greater than 3,000 IU (international units) per day, but there are reports of toxicity at doses greater than 1,200 units. Since vitamin E can be using to "thin the blood" based on its platelet mechanism, caution is advised when used with aspirin and other supplements, such as ginkgo and essential oils. Unless you are specifically prescribed higher doses, the appropriate amount of vitamin E to be taken daily is 400 IU.

Q. Is a good one-a-day vitamin all that is necessary? I have numb toes. Do I need more of a specific vitamin?

A. Well, it would be interesting to know why you have numb toes; a physician and/or podiatrist should be seen. Are you hypoglycemic or diabetic? If you have a history of unstable blood sugar, your numb toes may be a sign of neuropathy, a condition of numbness and tingling in the extremities, especially the feet. Even if you do not have a history of diabetes, it would be wise to have your glucose levels checked and even perhaps go for a glucose tolerance test. In any case, alpha lipoic acid has been shown to be effective in some neuropathies. Because this nutrient has a very short half-life—meaning that it does not last long in the bloodstream—it is better to take the 300-mg timed-release tablets that will provide coverage for up to 12 hours. Jarrow Formulas® makes a 300-mg timed-release tablet, and the suggested dose for neuropathy would be one pill twice a day. As far as a one-a-day supplement is concerned, it is wiser to take a few pills throughout the day to maximize absorption of all nutrients. If you are one of those individuals who will forget to take the afternoon and evening doses, then take a high-quality one-a-day such as VM75 by Solgar®. Other established and high-quality supplement manufacturers are in business that may also offer a good one-a-day.

Treating Conditions with Nutritional Supplements

You're on the Air...
Q. With the many recommendations concerning vitamins and supplements that are good for the heart, how does one determine the correct regimen for a specific condition?

A. This is a difficult question. I think vitamins and herbs should be prescribed for individual needs, based on the disease or condition. To determine a specific vitamin regimen, a physician must complete a thorough history and physical exam as well as study a blood profile analysis. It is important for the physician to discuss with the patient the dosages of prescription drugs already being taken by the patient. In some cases, certain vitamin levels can be measured, as in vitamin D, B_{12}, and folic acid. Simply put, there is no exact formula for specific dosages.

Q. I am 30 pounds overweight and I carry my weight in my abdomen. What would you recommend I do to lose the weight in this section of my body?

A. Weight in the midsection of the abdomen is a clear indication of unstable blood sugar levels (insulin resistance). I would recommend obtaining a 5-hour glucose tolerance test, with fasting, ½-hour, 1-hour, and 2-hour insulin levels assessed. This would indicate if you are a prediabetic and have insulin resistance. Insulin is a fat hormone. Based on the results, you would need a low-carbohydrate lifestyle with a moderate amount of good fats and less saturated fats. Any weight loss should be accompanied by an exercise program as outlined by your health care practitioner. People who carry their weight in their abdomen are more likely to suffer from heart disease than people who carry their weight proportionately, even if overweight. A potbelly is also a sign of stress. When I see patients who carry their weight in their midsection I know immediately that I am dealing with a person with high levels of cortisol, the hormone secreted by the adrenal glands. People with high cortisol levels also have insulin resistance, which means their bodies don't recognize the insulin that is being secreted by the pancreas, leading to increased sugar cravings; weight gain in the midsection; and often irritability, anxiety, and depression.

The best way to approach this is to cut back on the amount of sugars and refined carbohydrates you consume. Completely eliminate candy, cake, cookies, and muffins. Switch from white bread to hearty 9-grain bread that contains nuts and seeds, and eat that only in moderation. In addition, load up on vegetables and salads, and get high-quality sources of protein such as wild Alaskan salmon, tilapia, omega-3-enriched eggs, and organically fed chicken and turkey. Also eat nuts, seeds, and fruits, especially those low in sugars, such as berries and apples. If you have especially strong cravings for sugar and carbohydrates, you may want to try chromium picolinate. Start with 200 micrograms (mcg or μm) upon arising and on an empty stomach. If you feel as if you need more, you can safely increase to 600 mcg per day. I find that Longevity Nutritionals® provides an excellent product called GlucoStable™, designed to reduce sugar cravings and aid in stabilizing blood glucose levels. It will help make the transition easier for you. Chromium also helps to convert stored fat into energy and to lower cholesterol levels, so you will be getting the benefit of those as well.

This answer would not be complete without mentioning the importance of exercise. *It is literally the most important thing you can do for your health.* Just 30 minutes four times a week can go a long way toward improving your health. Studies show that people who begin an exercise program can decrease insulin resistance by up to 25% in as little as two weeks' time. This would be a vital addition to your weight loss and heart health lifestyle.

Q. Are there vitamins to help with an underactive thyroid?

A. Tyrosine and phenylalanine are two amino acids that stimulate thyroid function and have been shown to be very effective. Using kelp tablets has also been effective for nourishing the thyroid. That being said, I would not recommend that patients endeavor to treat underactive thyroid on their own. Taking thyroid-stimulating supplements incorrectly can lead to heart palpitations, insomnia, hair loss, and anxiety. It is best to seek out the counsel of a licensed and knowledgeable practitioner.

Q. What vitamins and supplements can be used in dealing with fatigue, without the harsh and somewhat addictive effects of using caffeine?

A. Before I go to supplements, allow me to discuss lifestyle modifications and how that can impact fatigue. When I see patients who are tired and fatigued, I always inquire about their diet. What foods are they eating? Do they grab a bagel on their way to work and then reach for a couple of pizza slices for lunch? Do they get adequate amounts of vegetables? What are their protein sources? All of this is important because stamina and energy begins with the foods we choose to eat. I would suggest that you begin your day with some protein, such as with a couple of eggs. Add diced asparagus and onions to that and you've got a nutritious omelet that will allow you to feel satisfied without the brain-numbing effects of refined carbohydrates. You will enjoy greater vitality, mental clarity and decreased hunger. So, cut back on the sugars and simple carbohydrates and load up on vegetables, fish, and chicken; add some beans and other legumes, as well as nuts and seeds, and you'll have the staples of an energy-boosting diet.

Of course, you would also benefit from a little bit of exercise. Start off slowly with some walking or perhaps easy yoga postures to get your body moving, eventually incorporating more cardiovascular work, such as jogging or swimming. Regular exercise is a wonderful way to stay energized throughout the day. It also helps improve mood and control cravings. Regular exercise can also improve the quality and quantity of sleep, which, in turn, will go a long way toward improving energy levels.

With regard to supplements, I would normally recommend B-complex vitamins. They are available in a variety of potencies. Patients suffering with fatigue often benefit by taking low doses more often throughout the day, rather than in one big dose. B-complex vitamins are water soluble, so whatever your body does not absorb gets moved out through the urine, turning it a bright yellow. I would also consider ginseng or ashwagandha, adaptogenic herbs that have been shown to improve energy levels, improve immune function, and help manage stress levels. Adaptogenic herbs help the body adapt to specific conditions or deficiencies. Benefits can be seen within one to two weeks. Another beneficial supplement is cordyceps, a Chinese mushroom that can help fight fatigue and boost energy levels as well.

Q. Are there vitamins to help with an overactive thyroid?

A. Unfortunately, not. There are foods you can try, such as tofu and other soy products and cruciferous vegetables (cabbage, kale, broccoli, Brussels sprouts, and cauliflower). It has been demonstrated in some studies that these foods will suppress thyroid function. Also, flax seed oil in high doses may inhibit an overactive thyroid.

Q. What vitamins should I take that are essential for good cardiac health and what role does iron play?

A. The organ that is most responsible for our longevity is the heart. For this reason alone, I test and treat for other risk indicators, besides the conventional cholesterol panel of tests. These Longevity Risk Factors™ include homocysteine, C-reactive protein, lipoprotein(a), fibrinogen, and insulin activity. There is no one diet that addresses all these concerns, presuming that you have a normal heart with no known blockages. The supplements used to prevent and maintain a healthy heart include

- Coenzyme Q$_{10}$ — 100–200 mg
- Magnesium — 600–800 mg
- L-Carnitine — 1,500–3,000 mg
- L-Taurine — 1,000–4,000 mg
- Essential Oils — 3,000–6,000 mg
- Tocotrienols — 200 mg
- B-complex — 50 mg
- —with folic acid — 2.5 mg
- Vitamin C — 2,000–4,000 mg

The herbs I consider to be most beneficial for a healthy heart include

- Hawthorne — up to 360 mg
- Ginkgo — 120–240 mg
- Garlic — 1,000–2,000 mg

The role of iron in the body is controversial. Some people do need iron, yet an excessive accumulation of iron is a risk factor for heart disease. For this reason, I usually recommend supplements that do not contain iron. In 1994, Antoni Dávalos, MD published an article revealing that high iron levels were associated with an increased risk of stroke. Studies have revealed that men with high concentrations of iron and copper in their bodies tend to oxidize the bad cholesterol faster and thereby develop an increased risk for atherosclerosis.

Q. Which food supplements help prevent arthritis and sinusitis?

A. Before discussing foods that can help prevent arthritis, I will discuss some supplements and herbs that can be used. Arthritis affects more than 45 million Americans and is still mismanaged in its treatment and care. Without discussing the difference between osteoarthritis and rheumatoid arthritis, I will list supplements that can be used instead of conventional prescription drugs with some success. Americans are fixated on the use of glucosamine and chondroitin sulfate for arthritis and cartilage problems. Methylsulfonylmethane, commonly known as MSM, can also be used to decrease inflammation, rebuild connective tissue, even increase hair and nail growth, as well as help the lungs. The supplement MSM is used in combination formulas with glucosamine and chondroitin; however, separate MSM doses of 6 to 9 grams might offer better results.

Cetyl myristoleate, which is a compound that combines the fatty acid myristoleic acid with cetyl alcohol, has been shown in European studies to lubricate joints, suppress inflammation, and even target the autoimmune reaction that may cause arthritis. The general course involves 16 to 18 grams over a six-week period. The ever-popular essential oils and gamma-linolenic acid (GLA, also a fatty acid) have traditionally been prescribed to patients with cardiovascular disease and those with arthritis. Published studies have shown that 1.4 grams of GLA reduces symptoms by 40% over the placebo-controlled studies.

Two herbs, ginger and turmeric, have been shown to decrease inflammation. Ginger is used as an antioxidant and an anti-inflammatory herb. Turmeric has been used in Chinese medicine to treat menstrual disorders, blood in the urine, and flatulence, and has also been used to decrease inflammation. In the last three years, studies have been done to demonstrate its anticancer and antioxidant actions. Studies have been done on its use in breast, colon, and kidney cancers. Studies are being done on the benefits of using turmeric in treating HIV/AIDS.

Foods to avoid if you have arthritis are the nightshade vegetables, such as tomatoes, potatoes, peppers, and eggplant. These nightshades contain solanine, a proinflammatory amino acid.

Sinusitis is a common problem, and many people resort to the use of antibiotics several times a year to combat infection. However, the frequent consumption of these antibiotics leads to yeast and fungal overgrowth, which creates an environment in the body where bugs can thrive, thereby leading to another infection.

For patients with a tendency to develop sinusitis, it is recommended that they avoid wheat, dairy, and sugar products. These foods provoke the excess production of mucus in the body, thereby creating moist breeding grounds for bacteria. I encourage patients to use substitutes, such as spelt and rice grains, instead of wheat (there are many fine companies out there making great breads with these alternative grains, which don't weaken the immune system in the way wheat does). I also suggest they try dairy substitutes, such as rice cheese or rice milk, instead of regular cow's dairy products. With regard to sugar, I try to get patients off the craving cycle that sugar inevitably leads to. Therefore, I do not recommend "fake sugar" substitutes, because these can enhance cravings. Instead I encourage them to satisfy a sweet tooth with fruit.

Beyond that, I find that daily nasal douching with a neti pot is the best preventive for sinusitis. Neti pots look like small teapots and are designed to thoroughly clear the nasal passages of mucus, dust, allergens, and bacteria. Two liquid solutions are recommended for use in a neti pot. The first and most common, is warm salt water. One-quarter teaspoon in 4 ounces of lukewarm water is the appropriate concentration, to be used upon arising. This is good for maintenance and prevention of infection. For those with an active infection, I would recommend you try a grapefruit seed extract that is prepared specifically for nasal douching and that is often sold with the neti pot.

Q. Which vitamins and minerals are good for increasing metabolism?

A. There are many nutrients that can be used to boost metabolism and aid in the conversion of fat into energy. One of the first ones to consider would be chromium picolinate, a mineral supplement that has shown to lessen cravings for sugar, help convert stored fat into energy, lower cholesterol, and stabilize blood glucose levels. The usefulness of this mineral cannot be overstated in its ability to help shed pounds. Another promising supplement is conjugated linoleic acid (CLA), a fatty acid supplement commonly found in grass-fed cows and dairy products; CLA helps convert stored fat into lean body tissue (muscle). The more muscle a person develops, the more efficiently they will burn fat. Patients on CLA report a decrease in dress size more so than pounds lost, since the fat that is being lost is being converted to the heavier muscle. This supplement also helps lower cholesterol, improve cognitive function, and stabilize glucose levels.

When looking for a fat-burning formula, look for ones that contain choline and inositol, nutrients that convert fat into energy and aid in detoxifying the liver. Most formulas will also add CoQ_{10}, vital for energy production in cells, as well as some amino acids like tyrosine and phenylalanine, which help to boost thyroid function, thereby boosting metabolism. However, you should use caution when taking L-phenylalanine and L-tyrosine, as they can both stimulate thyroid function. If you are on medication for hypothyroidism or have an overactive thyroid, the inclusion of these amino acids may lead to heart palpitations, excessive sweating, insomnia, and hair loss.

Green tea also has thermogenic (metabolism-boosting) properties so I always recommend patients drink green tea when looking to lose weight. This is a simple and inexpensive way to boost metabolism and get the added benefit of green tea's cancer-fighting potential, cholesterol-lowering properties, and antioxidant effects.

Q. Are there vitamins that help to prevent or delay Alzheimer's disease?

A. Alzheimer's disease is named after the physician Alois Alzheimer, who discovered unusual properties in the brain of a female patient. The findings were called *senile plaques*. We know that this is a chronic condition with no cure. There are two conventional medications on the market to stop the progression. One is Aricept® and the other is Namenda®. We currently do not know the cause of Alzheimer's disease. There are many speculations. We search for heavy metal intoxication as one potential cause.

There are some vitamins and herbs that help Alzheimer's disease. They include ginkgo, vitamin E, flavonoids, phosphatidyl choline, and phosphatidyl serine. One of the best nutrients to take for the prevention and support of Alzheimer's is acetyl-L-carnitine. This nutrient helps promote acetylcholine, a neurotransmitter responsible for concentration, memory, and recall. In addition to acetyl-L-carnitine, phosphatidyl serine has shown some promise in helping patients with Alzheimer's. Nicotinamide adenine dinucleotide (NADH), a coenzyme that energizes the brain, has also been used for the prevention of Alzheimer's and Parkinson's diseases.

Another important antioxidant, glutathione, has been used as a treatment and a preventive for Alzheimer's disease. It is difficult for the body to absorb glutathione when taken orally. Alternatively, a patient can consider taking NAC (N-acetyl cysteine), which is converted in the liver to glutathione. The preferred mode of delivery to the body is intravenously. This can be done either by a continuous intravenous infusion or by an intravenous "push" every 15 minutes.

Q. Is there a vitamin to increase my sexual drive?

A. There has been much research done on finding a sex-enhancing herb, or supplement to improve libido. They have been called *sexual rejuvenators*. However, none has been proven effective to date. Two herbs that have been studied are Siberian ginseng and sarsaparilla. Sarsaparilla contains a testosterone-like substance that can enhance arousal in men. Damiana is another herb that may be useful because it increases blood flow to the genital area.

An amino acid, L-arginine, has been used to increase blood flow in coronary arteries as well as penile and clitoral arteries, working in ways similar to Viagra® or Levitra®, although not as quickly. Caution should be used when taking arginine because it is a fuel for bacteria and viruses, including herpes, in the body and should only be used after ruling out any sort of infection that could be causing inflammation. It would be wise to get your C-reactive protein checked, which is a marker for inflammation and infection in the body. Anything over 0.5 would be a sign of some sort of infection, in which case, you would not be a candidate for arginine.

Other nutrients that are beneficial are zinc, a mineral that helps with the function of the prostate gland. Also, vitamin E can be helpful because it improves circulation. Other herbs, such as ginkgo and *Avena sativa,* have been used to help with erectile dysfunction.

Q. Are there vitamins, supplements, or nutritional strategies I should be aware of for improving cardiac health?

A. Section II in this book centers on vitamin supplements and herbs to promote a healthy heart. Every person should take healthy heart supplements. They include CoQ_{10}, essential oils, vitamin E, carnitine, taurine, and magnesium. There are many supplement formulas available that help to lower cholesterol naturally. Look for formulas that contain policosanols, gugulipids, red yeast rice, and niacin. A good high-potency formula, provided by Longevity Nutritions® called Cardio L™, is recommended because of its policosanol/beta-sitosterol concentrations. Another nutrient, lecithin, helps emulsify fat, thus making it easier for fat to be removed from the body and thereby helping to lower cholesterol. Lecithin is available in capsules and granules and should be taken after meals. Lecithin also has shown to be effective for weight loss.

Green tea extracts are often included in cholesterol-lowering formulas because of its thermogenic properties. If green tea extract is not in your formula, it would be wise to include this extract to your supplement protocol for its ability to lower cholesterol by up to 15% in some studies. It also helps prevent blockages in the arteries and has been shown to inhibit certain types of cancer.

But, as I tell all my patients, it is unwise to rely solely on supplements or medications when attempting to lower cholesterol. It cannot be overstated how important diet is in regards to a healthy cholesterol level. Often just by making simple adjustments to diet, you can manage cholesterol with minimal supplemental support.

It is vitally important to include exercise in your daily health regimen in order to protect your heart from disease. Ideally, you should be getting 30 to 45 minutes of exercise daily; however, four days per week is still very helpful. It doesn't have to be anything strenuous like aerobics or running. Simply walking at a brisk pace—during which you are increasing your heart rate but are not getting so winded that you cannot maintain a conversation—would be adequate. Another wonderful way to get exercise is to begin a yoga routine. If you are not able to attend a class, get a tape that you can follow at home, and try to do it four or five times a week. This is a wonderful way to improve circulation, build strength, and, most importantly for heart health, manage stress levels. Stress lands in the heart and if you don't engage in some sort of stress management activity, it can lead to heart disease.

Q. Can there be any benefit to taking vitamins for someone who has smoked for the past 60 years?

A. Absolutely! Unfortunately, 60 years is a long time to be smoking with regularity, but there is no time like the present for quitting and there are many nutritional supplements that would benefit an ex-smoker. To begin with, it would be wise to take a high-potency multivitamin/mineral supplement, one that would require you to take four to six pills a day. This is a great way to ensure that you are absorbing all of the nutrients in the supplement, rather than taking a one a day, which can potentially inhibit the proper absorption of all the nutrients contained by their competing for absorption. A good high-potency multiple would be Life Force Multi™ by Source Naturals®, and for an ex-smoker I would recommend you take 4 tablets daily in divided doses. I would also suggest that you take a green plant powder that aids in detoxification. Greens First® is an excellent green powder that includes chlorella, spirulina, spinach, milk thistle, and other green vegetables to help aid in detoxification. One scoop three times a day in water on an empty stomach for one month would be good to start. After that, decrease to two scoops daily. Another vital nutrient for ex-smokers would be N-acetyl-cysteine, an amino acid that aids in detoxification of the lungs and liver. It is also a precursor to glutathione, the most powerful antioxidant in the body. Take 500 mg three times a day on an empty stomach. And finally, it would be wise to include extra vitamin C with bioflavonoids to your protocol. Smokers tend to deplete vitamin C levels by up to 30 mg per cigarette! If you've been smoking for 60 years and not supplementing with vitamin C, then you will certainly benefit from taking a little extra than what is found in a multiple vitamin.

Supplements for Male and Female Health

You're on the Air...
Q. What healthy foods and supplements will produce better muscle mass for someone who is either beginning to work out or getting back to working out after a long period of not exercising?

A. The best food sources for promoting muscle mass would be protein. I recommend the leaner sources of protein, such as fish, eggs, chicken, and turkey. Of course, balance the protein with vegetables and complex carbohydrates, such as moderate amounts of brown rice, multigrain breads, and sweet potatoes. Include nuts and seeds and moderate amounts of fruits.

An appropriate food supplement for building muscle mass would be one of the whey protein powders. With their broad spectrum of amino acids and enhanced absorption, this is the best source of supplemental protein for building muscle mass. Take it after a workout to improve recovery time. It can also be blended with a combination of fruits for a treat-like smoothie.

Ginseng has also been used to enhance recovery time, thereby improving muscle mass. When taken daily for maximum effects, this herb has the added benefits of improving energy levels, enhancing immune function, and managing stress.

Branched-chain amino acids (leucine, isoleucine, and valine) are also popular among body builders for their ability to maintain muscle mass and prevent muscle protein breakdown during exercise. These essential amino acids are called *essential* because they cannot be manufactured in the body and must be obtained through dietary sources, such as dairy and meat products. These amino acids are also available together in supplement form.

Q. What is your opinion about coffee? I feel that I need it to jump-start my workout. I cannot seem to get going without it. What are your thoughts?

A. I have a lot of opinions about coffee. I secretly love it and wish it was one of the power foods that help prevent degenerative disease. Despite sporadic findings touting its dubious health-promoting effects, this will never be. Coffee will never be on the must-consume list of the best foods to eat for your health. Besides coffee's obvious deleterious effects, such as anxiety, irritability, and sleeplessness, coffee is a toxic, acid-forming beverage that should be consumed infrequently. It is hard on the liver and promotes acidosis in the gut, affecting digestion and absorption of nutrients. Acidity in the body weakens the immune system, increases stress, and promotes aging. This widely used beverage also affects brain function, with studies showing that prolonged coffee consumption has been linked to depression. A single cup of coffee depletes serotonin levels for up to ten hours! This means that the beneficial calming effects of serotonin are lost to you for ten hours. What this in turn promotes is higher stress levels and increased cravings for sugar.

The reason coffee kick-starts your workout is because it promotes the release of dopamine and norepinephrine in the brain, neurotransmitters that help with focus and concentration, at the same time producing adrenaline. Exercise in and of itself requires the use of adrenaline, and this combination can eventually lead to burn out. Instead of coffee, try switching to tea. Although tea also contains caffeine, black tea contains only one-half the amount of caffeine and green tea contains less than one-fourth the amount of caffeine, as compared with coffee. Either of these choices will also help in maintaining a healthy cholesterol level and improve circulation. Green tea has been shown to decrease the incidence of developing cancers and has also exhibited thermogenic (metabolism-boosting) properties. You can also try one of the adaptogenic herbs like ashwagandha or ginseng. These help boost energy levels and combat fatigue when taken regularly. They will also enhance immune function.

Q. What vitamins are essential for men's health?

A. There are multiple supplements and herbs than men can take to lead a better life. Two of the most important problems that affect men are benign prostatic hyperplasia and low libido. Americans spend more than $4 billion annually in managing the benign enlargement of the prostate gland, both medically and surgically. However, with a change in paradigm, there are increasing amounts of money being spent on alternative treatments for this condition. The most important supplements are saw palmetto extracts; amino acids such as alanine and glycine; the minerals zinc, selenium, and manganese; and vitamin E. To increase a man's sex drive or for those who suffer from impotence, there are supplements to help. Men would also benefit from taking the mineral zinc and the carotenoid lycopene to help in the prevention of benign prostatic hyperplasia. Abundant in tomatoes, especially cooked tomatoes, lycopene is often recommended as an adjunct in the treatment of prostate cancer.

With the use of conventional prescription drugs such as Viagra® for impotence, the role of supplements in this area has diminished. The most important supplements include high doses of arginine (an amino acid); two herbs—ginkgo and ginseng; and androstenedione can be used. I would like to also mention yohimbine, which has been used traditionally in Africa as a male aphrodisiac. It has been studied for its effectiveness in male erectile dysfunction, and diabetes. Because this herb has many toxic side effects, such as hypertension, kidney problems, and tachycardia, it should be used with caution.

Because many men suffer from stress and fatigue, I would also consider an adaptogenic herb like rhodiola root or ginseng. Known for their immunity-enhancing properties and their ability to boost energy while managing stress, these herbs would be a safer alternative to prescription stress management medications such as Valium®. All people would benefit from including omega-3 oils in the diet to ensure healthy cholesterol levels, decrease the clotting factor in blood (fibrinogen), and to prevent inflammation. Since many men are prone to arthritis and other inflammatory conditions as they age, a good way to begin to combat that is through the consumption of omega-3 oils.

Q. What are the most effective supplements for a middle-aged man to take on a daily basis?

A. Enzymatic Therapy® makes a multiple vitamin/mineral/herbal supplement for men over 50 that is geared toward their needs. This supplement contains nutrients to protect the prostate gland and support heart health. It also provides the necessary nutrients for men over 50.

Q. At what age should a man or woman take saw palmetto?

A. Saw palmetto has been used for centuries by Native Americans in the treatment of urinary tract disturbances and as a tonic. It is a plant that is native to the West Indies and to the U.S. Atlantic coastal states. It has also been heralded as an aphrodisiac.

There are numerous results that support its efficacy and clinical application in the treatment of benign prostatic hyperplasia (BPH) by inhibiting the conversion of testosterone to dihydrotestosterone, the latter of which causes the gland to grow larger than necessary. Approximately 50 to 60% of men aged 40 to 59 years old develop BPH, so it is suggested that men begin treatment with saw palmetto at this time.

Studies have compared its effectiveness to a commonly prescribed conventional drug, Proscar®, with saw palmetto achieving better results. It is one of the few herbs that multiple double-blind clinical trials have studied. The recommended dose is 160 mg twice a day of a standardized extract containing 85 to 95% fatty acids and sterols.

Saw palmetto is predominantly used for males, but it has been shown to exert a tonic effect on the uterus, vaginal walls, and ovaries, lessening tenderness, dryness, and pain associated with menopause. Saw palmetto has also been shown to diminish unwanted facial hair in women. Women interested in using saw palmetto to treat any of these symptoms should begin by taking a tea form of saw palmetto several times a day. If that proves insufficient, then try a standardized extract, containing 85 to 95% fatty acids in a 160-mg capsule once a day.

Q. What are the most effective supplements for a middle-aged woman to take on a daily basis?

A. Enzymatic Therapy® is a professional vitamin line that makes high-quality supplements for every stage of life. They make a combination supplement specifically for females over 45 that is appropriate for the challenges faced by women over that age. This supplement is enriched with herbs and vitamins that stabilize hormone fluctuations associated with menopause and are produced iron free, because most women do not need to supplement iron after menopause.

Q. My hair started falling out about a year ago, so I cut it off, but now it is not growing back at all. It seems that even more is falling out. What would be the best vitamin for me to take so that it will grow back healthier and longer?

A. Before you begin with a supplement protocol, it would be wise for you to have your thyroid checked, specifically, your thyroid-stimulating hormone (TSH) levels. Thinning hair is often a sign of impaired thyroid function: both under-and oversecretion. Hypothyroidism is easily treated with natural thyroid extracts and once this is corrected, hair begins to grow back properly. That being said, there are many supplements on the market that have been shown to promote hair growth and strength. I would begin with a supplement with adequate amounts of B vitamins, especially biotin. Biotin supplementation can improve the quality and quantity of hair. Other important nutrients include silica or horsetail, minerals, and pantothenic acid and inositol. I also love the benefits of flax seed. It makes hair feel and look healthier, fuller, and with greater shine. Take one tablespoonful per hundred pounds of body weight for best results.

Q. My wife is 39 years old. She needs something for energy and libido. What do you suggest?

A. Stress is a huge factor that impacts women in regards to their libido. My questions to you would be, "how many responsibilities and challenges does your wife face in a day? Does she work during the day and then come home and care for kids, cook dinner, and then clean the house?" If this sounds like a typical day for her, then it is reasonable to think that her lack of interest in sex could have something to do with exhaustion. She may simply be tired. If this is the case, perhaps getting a babysitter for the kids so that you can enjoy a night out alone may be helpful. Making one night a week "date night," when you can go out as a couple and enjoy each other without the burden of kids and responsibilities, may be very helpful in relaxing your wife enough to get her in the mood. Keep in mind that if there are communication problems between you and your wife, those, too, could be a reason for her lack of interest.

Another approach to discovering why your wife may have a low sex drive is to have her thyroid function tested. Often, hypothyroidism affects libido, so I would suggest that she have her thyroid checked in order to rule that out.

In regards to supplements that can be used, damiana is an herb that is also known as the "woman's sexuality herb." It is a wonderful herb for supporting and enhancing sexuality and arousal. It may be used as soon as two hours before sexual activity, although for best results it should be used daily. Other herbs that may be beneficial include gotu-kola, Siberian ginseng, and sarsaparilla.

Arginine is an amino acid that has shown to enhance arousal in the same way that Viagra® does although not as quickly or as intensely. It needs to be taken daily for maximum results. It helps enhance circulation to the genital area, thus facilitating arousal and climax. Caution should be used with arginine as it is a fuel for bacteria and viruses that promote inflammation in the body, so it would be recommended that you have your C-reactive protein level checked. C-reactive protein is a marker for inflammation and infection in the body, and, if it is elevated, arginine should be avoided.

Q. Is there a reliable resource that will tell me exactly which vitamins and minerals are in vegetables and fruits and how they can be used healthwise?

A. A good resource for this information is the book *Power Plants*, by Kim O'Neill, PhD and Byron Murray, PhD. It includes several chapters on the nutritional value of fruits and vegetables as well as other valuable information, such as what to eat in order to avoid particular illnesses, such as heart disease and cancer.

Q. Can you provide me with a list of vitamins and supplements that should not be combined with conventional medications?

A. This list is endless and cannot be addressed in this book. I suggest you consult the *PDR® for Nutritional Supplements* and the *PDR® for Herbal Medicines, third edition,* for interactions, as well as seeing a practitioner familiar with integrative medicine. It is important that you educate yourself on potential interactions before beginning any vitamin or herbal supplementation to ensure they will not interfere with any medication you have been prescribed.

Section II.

Herbs for the Heart

Herbs for the Heart

There is nothing new about herbal therapy. It promotes recovery, wellness, and health. Throughout the history of the world, there have been references made to the power of healing through herbs. For instance, we can find this written in the Bible, and among the teachings of traditional Chinese medicine and Native American Indians.

The interesting point to note is that medicine has its foundations in the use of herbs. As a cardiologist, I always point to the foxglove plant, from which the conventional drug digoxin is derived. Digoxin is used in conventional cardiology to treat atrial fibrillation (an arrhythmia) and in congestive heart failure.

Herbal medicine practitioners believe in the philosophy of working through the whole body, yet there are certain herbs that have been used for certain conditions. Common examples of this are valerian for anxiety and insomnia, St. John's wort for depression, hawthorn for the heart, echinacea for common colds, and black cohosh for menopausal symptoms. The list goes on and on.

It is estimated that more than 60% of all health care consumers in the United States take some form of herbal or "natural" products. These may be taken alone or combined with a conventional medication. The therapeutic value of some of the herbs has not been studied or been proven effective, but the promotion and marketing strategies of some herbal products has made their use widespread.

The purpose of answering some of your most frequently asked questions about herbs and some of their benefits in disease is trifold.

1. Some of these products can interact with conventionally prescribed medications.

2. Some herbal products may be harmful to some patients and their medical conditions.

3. Some of the consumers who use herbal therapies and supplements as alternative approaches never mention this fact to their conventional doctors.

You're on the Air...
Q. What is the normal pulse rate for women?

A. The normal pulse rate, or heart rate, is 60 to 100 beats per minute. The term *bradycardia* refers to a pulse of fewer than 60 beats/min, whereas the term *tachycardia* is a pulse rate greater than 100 beats/min. The use of specific herbs for arrhythmias will be discussed in Section III of this book, but I will introduce some herbal remedies for arrhythmias at this time. The common heart tonic herbs include hawthorn, motherwort, night blooming cactus, scotch broom, lily of the valley, and bugleweed.

Hawthorn is the most commonly used herb for circulatory problems. It acts to dilate the blood vessels, thus decreasing blood pressure, and improves and strengthens the contractions of the heart, as does foxglove. Some of the conditions that hawthorn has been used to treat are hypertension, congestive heart failure, angina pectoris, and Buerger's disease. The antiviral and antioxidant effects of some hawthorn plant species were studied in 2002. Its cardiovascular effects were discussed in peer-reviewed articles from Germany in 2000. One study examined its effect compared with placebo at 600-mg doses in patients with congestive heart failure, and favorable results were obtained for those who took hawthorn compared with the placebo group.

Hawthorn should be used with caution in patients taking conventional medications such as beta-blockers (atenolol, lopressor, etc.) and cardiac glycosides (digoxin, which is derived from the foxglove plant). Hawthorne may increase the effect of some of the conventionally prescribed antidepressants, such as Celexa®, Lexapro®, Zoloft®, and so on.

Q. Is garlic the only blood-thinning supplement available, or are there other supplements that you could recommend?

A. Garlic is a member of the lily family, and records indicate that it had been used almost 4,000 years ago. Even the great doctor and philosopher, Hippocrates and Aristotle, respectively, had uses for garlic. There is a wide range of well-documented and researched effects of garlic. In addition to the anti-platelet action (the blood-thinning effect), garlic has been used to treat infections ranging from fungi to worms. There is a large amount of evidence to support the beneficial effects of garlic in the prevention of cancer. Garlic protects against heart disease and stroke by interfering in the development of plaque in blood vessel walls. These are the anti-platelet effects of garlic. We do know that excessive clumping of platelets plays a role in the development of plaque. In 1991, Kiesewetter compared the effects of garlic in one group versus a group given placebo. Platelet aggregation disappeared in the garlic group.

Also noted were decreases in blood pressure and cholesterol levels. Garlic will also interfere in the fibrinolytic activity in the body; thus, it will cause the blood to be thinner. When a patient is taking garlic, I recommend measuring the clotting factors, including fibrinogen. This is an important point because fibrinogen, a protein involved in the clotting system, is an independent risk factor for heart disease. It is one of the Longevity Risk Factors for heart disease.

Other natural therapies to help with anti-platelet action or in thinning the blood are omega-3 oils, bromelain, and capsicum. Bromelain is used extensively in Europe to reverse the symptoms of heart disease. It is also used in keeping platelets from clumping or sticking to each other, thus causing a blockage or plaque.

Q. Could you provide me with nutritional strategies to improve circulation and especially to the arms and legs? I have been experiencing tingling and numbness in my

extremities, and I would like to know what I could do to combat that.

A. Poor circulation to the hands and legs can be another indication of hardening of the arteries, technically referred to as *atherosclerosis*. Pain in the lower extremities upon exertion, such as walking, is termed *claudication*. A definitive diagnosis should be sought to determine the exact degree of arterial narrowing. In some cases and for severe narrowing, a stent might need to be placed. For lesions or blockages less than 70 to 80%, there are herbs and supplements that can alleviate the pain. Four herbs come to mind for improving circulation: ginkgo, mistletoe, hawthorn, and linden. One herb, horse chestnut, is used in the treatment of venous insufficiency and varicose veins. The use of any of the herbs above with conventional medications, such as aspirin, Plavix®, and Coumdin®, can cause an interaction with the possibility of an increased risk for bleeding.

Q. Can my skipped heartbeats, or palpitations, be related to anxiety?

A. Anxiety and stress can cause palpitations or skipped heartbeats. As a cardiologist, I would want to perform an echocardiogram and a 24-lead electrocardiogram to ensure that there are no pathologic causes to the palpitations, such as heart valve disease or arrhythmias.

There are herbal remedies that can be used for anxiety. The most common nervous system tonics or relaxants that can be used include valerian, skullcap, and mistletoe. I have found the most effective combination is skullcap and valerian, which can be drunk as a tea. The only negative drawback of this mixture is the taste, which is not very pleasant. Valerian is used to treat anxiety, insomnia, and restlessness. It may increase the effects of other conventionally prescribed drugs, so avoid combined use. Since it can cause elevations in liver enzymes, I would have your doctor regularly check your liver enzymes.

Q. I have a very high C-reactive protein (CRP) level (almost 10), and heart disease runs in my family. I would like to know what I could take to decrease my CRP and reduce my risk for heart disease.

A. C-reactive protein levels reflect inflammation in the body. With regard to CRP, there are two types of this blood test. One is the general CRP, which indicates overall body inflammation. I concentrate on the second type of CRP, known as the *high-sensitivity*, or *cardiac CRP*. This test indicates inflammation and possible infection of the coronary arteries. I identify this risk factor as one of the Longevity Risk Factors™, which go beyond cholesterol testing. The Longevity Risk Factors™ are discussed in Section III. Cardiac CRP, when elevated, has been linked to an increased risk of cardiovascular disease. As mentioned in Section II, a search for the possible infections that can cause an increase in the cardiac CRP should be conducted.

There are two herbs that I use that can reduce inflammation. Turmeric and ginger have been efficacious in reducing inflammation associated with arthritis and other joint diseases. There are studies that note its effect on platelet aggregation. This is important because increased platelet aggregation can lead to clot formation.

Ginger has been used for nausea, vomiting, and migraine. I would rather use feverfew for prevention and treatment of migraines. Turmeric has traditionally been used in Chinese medicine to treat menstrual disorders. I have used turmeric to treat a variety of diseases, including gastrointestinal disorders, arthritis, and even HIV/AIDS. It does exhibit anticancer and antioxidant effects. Since turmeric can interact with anticoagulant drugs, such as Coumadin and aspirin, it should be used with the guidance of a physician. To decrease inflammation, I combine these herbs with vitamin C and bioflavonoids.

Q. If I take a medication called atenolol for my blood pressure, can I also take hawthorn?

A. The medication called atenolol is a class of cardiovascular medications called *beta-blockers*. This class is used to treat both abnormal hearts and blood pressure. Without the guidance of a health care practitioner, I would caution against using the herb hawthorn with a beta-blocker. Hawthorne provides us with one of the best heart tonics for the heart and circulatory system.

Q. My doctor has told me that I have borderline high blood pressure. On every visit he wants to put me on a conventional medicine. Are there are any herbs that can lower my blood pressure?

A. Hypertension is a preventable disease. I will discuss other questions relating to supplements for hypertension in Section III. Patients with hypertension are four times more likely to experience a major cardiovascular event, such as heart attack or stroke.

The treatment strategy is to lower the future risk of cardiovascular damage. Lifestyle modification with weight reduction; sodium restriction; and discontinuation of nicotine, alcohol, and caffeine should first be implemented. There is a role for conventional prescribed medication if the blood pressure elevations have already affected your renal system (kidneys).

With the help of a skilled and licensed practitioner, taking herbs is a safe way to strengthen your heart. These herbs can be used as dried extracts (capsules), tinctures (alcohol based), and even teas. If a tea is used, it must be consumed three to four times a day and must steep for at least 10 minutes for leaves and flowers and even longer for those derived from roots.

Some of these herbs include hawthorn, linden flowers, passion flower, and cramp bark. Since hawthorn has already been discussed, I will now discuss some of the other herbs.

Passion flower has been used to treat anxiety and insomnia as well as nervous tachycardia. It has in the past been studied and researched in the treatment of Parkinson's disease. I have found that these herbs, although effective, should be used with other supplements to decrease blood pressure, such as taurine, carnitine, magnesium. and CoQ_{10}. Since blood pressure reductions respond to a diuretic effect, the herb dandelion leaf can be used. Dandelion is a weed found throughout the world. Dandelion has been used experimentally as an anti-tumor agent. Some other herbs that have a profound effect on blood pressure and should be used with caution include lily of the valley and night blooming cactus. Both of these herbs are also used to treat atrial fibrillation, which is discussed in Section III.

Section III.

Addressing Specific Cardiac Conditions with Integrative Approaches

Cardiovascular Disease and the Use of Supplements and Herbs

We know that cardiovascular disease is the leading cause of death in developed countries. I have been caring for patients with heart disease for more than 10 years, and during the course of my career, especially in the last 5 years, I have heard the same questions over and over. Everyone wants to know if there are any supplements and herbs that can be taken to help maintain a healthy heart. In the same breath, people want to know if there are any supplements or herbs that can replace some of the conventionally prescribed drugs they are taking.

Every 33 seconds, an American dies of cardiovascular disease, which accounts for greater than 1 million deaths annually. Statistics show that every 22 seconds an American suffers a heart attack and every 60 seconds an American dies from one or more cardiovascular conditions. Among the conditions included in this section are:

1. Coronary artery disease
2. Hyperlipidemia
3. Arrhythmias
4. Valvular heart disease, cardiomyopathy, and congestive heart failure
5. Hypertension

This section will answer by disease some of your commonly asked questions.

Coronary Artery Disease

Conventional medicine believes that lowering your blood pressure and lipid levels with medication will lower your risk for having a heart attack or stroke. To some extent this is true; however, there are other answers.

There are more than 150 million visits to physicians' offices each year for high blood pressure. High blood pressure can lead to coronary artery disease. In most cases, the prescription pad comes out of the desk drawer and the doctor prescribes a conventional medication to lower the blood pressure. You have to ask yourself the question, "Why didn't my physician consider supplements over a conventional medication?" The supplements CoQ_{10}, taurine, and carnitine can be used to treat high blood pressure. Maybe your physician just doesn't know this.

Within the last two years, more than 701,000 coronary artery bypass surgeries were performed at astronomical costs. Most surgeries were done on men. However, there has been an increased death rate from heart disease among women over the last few years. Other invasive procedures, such as angioplasty and stent implantation, have been done at increasing numbers at additional costs to health care industries and to the patient.

For 2004, the total estimated cost of cardiovascular disease, including treatment and disability, adds up to greater than 270 billion dollars. Our aim should be on such preventive measures as stress reduction, weight reduction, dietary improvement, and quit-smoking programs. In addition, we should be placing emphasis on use of certain supplements and herbs to prevent heart disease. We should explore other alternative approaches to eliminating plaque in the coronary arteries, such as intravenous chelation and phosphatidyl choline therapies. Patients who are too old or medically unsuitable for bypass and other invasive procedures should consider a conventional therapy that is noninvasive, such as enhanced external counterpulsation (EECP®). This atraumatic treatment, which is provided for 1 hour/day for 35 days, has been approved by the FDA and is supported by the American College of Cardiology for treatment of coronary artery disease. I wish that more people could become aware of this conventional therapy. Currently, EECP is performed at more than 300 locations throughout the United States, as well as in Argentina, Canada, Colombia, France, Germany, India, Ireland, Israel, Italy, Japan, Saudi Arabia, Turkey, and the United Kingdom. Visit http://www.eecp.com/and elsewhere for more information.

When plaque or atherosclerosis develops in a coronary artery, the heart is deprived of oxygen-rich blood owing to a partially or totally clogged artery. The total blockage results in a heart attack, termed a *myocardial infarction*. A partially blocked artery may result in pain in the chest, known as *angina pectoris*.

Some of the heart attack warning signs include chest pain, shoulder pain, jaw pain, nausea, excessive sweating, and back pain. When the patient does not receive an adequate amount of oxygen-rich blood via a coronary artery, such symptoms can occur. However, heart attacks can appear without warning. There are some patients who have no symptoms and yet experience a heart attack. This can be referred to as *silent angina*, in which there is no pain in the chest but instead shortness of breath, numbness in the arm, and even dizziness.

With the rising numbers in loss of life and rising health care costs, it is imperative that we understand the risk factors for heart disease. The atherosclerotic plaque has historically been linked to inflammatory lesions. So what causes this inflammation? More recently, researchers have wondered what role this inflammation could play in the thinning of the cap that covers the plaque, plaque rupture, and clotting—all which can lead to heart attack and stroke.

Well-known and traditional risk factors for coronary artery disease include elevated stress levels, high blood pressure, physical inactivity, poor diet, and diabetes. In the past, the only clinical markers used were lipid levels, which include total cholesterol, low-density lipoproteins (LDL), high-density lipoproteins (HDL), and triglycerides.

Some other risk factors, such as homocysteine level, were suggested as early as 1969 but only recently have been extensively studied as risk factors for coronary artery disease. The one risk factor that must be sought after is the C-reactive protein (CRP). Cardiac CRP is a specific

Section III. Addressing Specific Cardiac Conditions with Integrative Approaches

marker for inflammation and infection of the coronary arteries. Studies have shown that increases in cardiac CRP are associated with a higher risk for coronary artery disease. This associated increase is independent of other risk factors. This means that despite normal lipid panel results you are still at risk for a heart attack.

There have been 20 or more different bacteria and viruses identified that can cause infection and inflammation. Some of these include mycoplasmal species, *Helicobacter pylori*, chlamydial species, herpes simplex viruses, *Nanobacterium sanguineum*, and cytomegalovirus. There are studies to correlate the increased risk of cardiovascular disease with mouth (periodontal) infections. Since there is a link between platelet sticking and CRP, there have been studies that demonstrate the control of fibrinogen (a clotting factor) and platelet sticking with nutrients such as omega-3 fatty acids.

There have been a number of questions asked regarding previous history of heart attack, stroke or invasive procedures, such as angioplasty and stent. This section will answer your most asked questions concerning supplements for the heart.

You're on the Air...
Q. I would like to remove plaque without having any surgery. My husband had a heart attack in 1999 and we both have eaten the same way for 38 years. I believe I am now experiencing the same signs that my husband had. I was nauseous and had pain in my jaw. I took a three-week leave and started to feel better. I am still concerned. Do you think it could have been my heart?

A. I first will address the latter part of the question. Signs and symptoms of decreased blood flow to the heart can be varied and individualized, from person to person. The classic sign that every individual knows is central chest pain that radiates down the left arm. Although this is classic angina pectoris, every patient has their own anginal (pain) equivalent. What I mean is that a patient can experience nausea, jaw pain, shoulder pain, pain down the right arm, and even back pain. One or more of those symptoms might be their anginal equivalent. Nausea can also be a sign of a heart attack and typically would involve the right coronary artery because that artery is above the diaphragm, near the stomach area.

Despite the fact that your pain was relieved after a medical leave is no reason not to have a cardiac work-up done. This would include an electrocardiogram (electrical tracing of the heart) and an echocardiogram (ultrasound of the heart). The echocardiogram will reveal any problems with your valves, particularly whether they are regurgitant (leaky when closed) or stenotic (too narrow when open). The other important information gathered from an echocardiogram is the patient's ejection fraction (pumping function of the heart). Based on the results of these tests in addition to a blood analysis of Longevity Risk Factors™, the doctor might also want a stress test.

The first part of your question was concerned with how to remove plaque without surgery. This question has been answered in multiple books. You didn't specify the location of the plaque; however, I will assume from your question you are referring to plaque within the coronary arteries. Plaque consists of cholesterol, calcium, other lipoproteins, and platelets. There is no wonder drug or procedure to remove plaque. Interventional procedures push the plaque against the arterial wall, as in angioplasty or stent implantation. There have been studies published since the 1960s on the cardiovascular benefits of chelation therapy. Chelation therapy using ethylenediaminetetraacetic acid (EDTA), as currently practiced appears to be safe, and there are many mechanisms postulated that are biologically plausible for the treatment of atherosclerosis.

The American College for Advancement in Medicine (ACAM) has trained over 7,000 physicians in the use of chelation therapy throughout the world. EDTA was first patented in 1939 and initially used and approved for lead intoxication. At that time, there were reports of its benefits in heart disease. In the 1950s, there was discussion regarding the benefits in removing unwanted calcium deposits, whereas other series of articles described symptomatic benefits in patients with angina pectoris. In the 1980s, Casdorph and Robinson provided improvements in both ejection fraction and ECGs, respectively. In the 1990s, Hancke described a study in which 39 out of 42 patients cancelled their surgery (either coronary artery surgery or amputation) after chelation therapy. So where are we in the year 2004? I do utilize chelation therapy for the treatment of atherosclerotic heart disease. Our chelation patients have reported a decrease in anginal symptoms (chest pain), improvement in exercise capability, improvement in peripheral vascular disease, and an increase in pain-free walking distances. They have either decreased or eliminated their need for bypass graft surgery and amputation for peripheral vascular disease.

EDTA is administered intravenously for between 1 and 3 hours depending on the patient's kidney function and the physician's clinical judgment. Frequency of treatment depends on the patient's disease, tolerance, and convenience. The usual number of chelation treatments ranges from 10 to 40. Serum blood tests for kidney function are carefully monitored in patients receiving EDTA. Along with the EDTA, the infusion contains trace minerals and vitamin C. In addition to the benefits of EDTA as a chelator to calcium and other metals, EDTA also can act as an antioxidant, it improves lipid metabolism, and it stimulates capillary blood flow. There are few side effects to EDTA. Some include local irritation, hypoglycemia, and hypocalcemia. Hypoglycemia is not seen if the patient follows dietary instructions before infusion therapy. An ongoing research project into EDTA therapy titled Trial to Assess Chelation Therapy (TACT) is being done by the National Institutes of Health.

This is only one method to remove plaque, assuming that the plaque is calcium in nature. We also utilize another infusion treatment called Plaquex® (phosphatidylcholine). The Plaquex program utilizes this essential phospholipid (lecithin) in the form of a series of infusions to clear blocked arteries. This phospholipid is derived from soybeans.

The most important effect of Plaquex is its remarkable ability to reduce deposits of plaque in the arterial wall. Clinical studies on animals indicate that treating relatively aged animals with Plaquex over an extended period of time increased their lifespan by 36%. Another important use of Plaquex is to increase male potency. It reverses the age-related changes in the lipid composition of vital organs and tissues, such as heart cells and red blood cells, by lipid exchange.

During the course of treatment, the patient's anginal symptoms disappear. Plaquex treatment shows marked improvement in patients with reduced blood flow to the brain, heart, and other vital organs, such as the kidneys, and to the extremities.

Prior to the therapy, important serum blood tests are taken. As with EDTA therapy, we encourage our patients to undergo a scan to determine the extent of calcium blockage in the coronary arteries and a CT-angiogram (a noninvasive angiogram of the coronary arteries). The Plaquex treatment is administered over a period of 60 to 80 minutes. A minimum of 20 Plaquex treatments are recommended; however, as with all programs in our practice, we individualize them. Occasionally, patients with a severe case of atherosclerosis can initially experience diarrhea, which can be controlled with conventional drugs, such as Imodium®. There also may be an increase in liver enzymes. There are some isolated reports of phlebitis (inflammation of a vein) at the infusion site.

Q. I feel OK. In February, I had a small heart attack. I am a 60-year-old white female with exceptional blood results. I have had my cardiac CRP and homocysteine checked, which are normal. What other blood tests should I have done?

A. A postmenopausal female with a known heart attack should have two other conventional blood tests. They are lipoprotein(a) and fibrinogen. Both are Longevity Risk Factors™ and are linked to coronary artery disease. Both of these risk factors are elevated in the postmenopausal patient. Both of these can be treated with nutrition and supplements. Fibrinogen (a clotting factor) can be treated with essential oils, bromelain, and vitamin E. Lipoprotein(a) can be decreased with vitamin C; two amino acids, proline and lysine; niacin; and coenzyme Q_{10}. The normal lipoprotein(a) level is less than 20. The statin drugs, which are commonly used to lower total cholesterol and LDL, have no effect on lowering lipoprotein(a).

Q. What vitamins, supplements, and nutritional strategies can you recommend for a patient after a six-vessel bypass who was left with an ejection fraction of 26% and recurrent thrombophlebitis with ulcers. This patient is my 57-year-old brother, who also has diabetes. He is also considering hyperbaric oxygen. What are some of your suggestions?

A. This patient has a diagnosis of coronary artery disease and has undergone heart bypass surgery. The pumping function of his heart is below normal. His diabetes is complicated with persistent inflammation and ulceration in the lower extremities.

Why does a 57-year-old man get a bypass? Other questions that I ask myself are, "Was his diabetes managed properly with nutrition and supplements; was his lipid panel elevated; and, most important, did he have other cardiac risk factors elevated prior to his surgery?" The risk factors that go beyond total cholesterol and the bad cholesterol include homocysteine, lipoprotein(a), fibrinogen, and cardiac CRP. All of these risk factors are determined and evaluated on a simple blood test. Some of these risk factors were identified as far back as 1969.

Hyperbaric oxygen therapy has been used for the treatment of chronic ulcers associated with diabetes. There are many wound-care centers in the United States that utilize hyperbaric oxygen therapies. The other approved conditions for the use of hyperbaric oxygen therapies have been acute stroke and chronic Lyme disease. There are other centers that utilize hyperbaric for the treatment of chronic fatigue syndrome, but there is no clinical or supporting evidence for this use.

Q. I am a 55-year-old white male with a family history of coronary artery disease. My father died at age 58. I want to prevent a heart attack. I have listened to you on the radio and take multiple supplements. Should I take an aspirin?

A. The typical doctor response is, "An aspirin a day helps keep the heart attack away." Aspirin is the most widely used medication, taken over 60 billion times per year worldwide for a variety of reasons. A baby aspirin, 81 mg, provides plenty of protection with very low risk of stomach and other bleeding. I would caution against the use of aspirin with high doses of such supplements as ginkgo, essential oils, and vitamin E. But remember, no pill can make up for the harm that comes from smoking, poor nutrition, and lack of exercise.

Q. There are many diets books I have read. I am more confused about the amount of carbohydrates I should use. When does the intake of carbohydrates become a problem in relation to my heart?

A. The National Academy of Sciences sets 130 grams of carbohydrates as the minimum daily level needed to fuel the brain. In the amount of food, that equates to two slices of whole-grain bread, a bowl of shredded wheat, a banana, an apple, and a cup of yogurt. Most Americans eat two to three times the minimum requirement. An increase in carbohydrates leads to a high triglyceride level, and thus a lower high-density lipoprotein (HDL) level (the good cholesterol). Triglycerides are a major risk factor of coronary artery disease and is also a risk factor for the development of insulin resistance and Type II diabetes. So there is a good reason to cut back on total carbohydrates and especially the highly processed carbohydrates. In regards to the diets you have been reading about, the beginning phases of some diets call for only 20 grams of carbohydrates, which is less than a sixth of the recommended daily allowance.

Q. Why is it important for me to exercise? I am not inactive, but what exactly does exercise do for an individual?

A. As a cardiologist I issue an exercise prescription to all my patients. I try to recommend an exercise that is easy, comfortable, and likable to the patient. Walking is the easiest for any individual, barring any physical restrictions as hip, back, and foot problems. Regular exercise improves mood, keeps the muscles toned, increases energy, improves sleep, and reduces the risk of obesity and heart disease. More than 70% of Americans are sedentary and truly miss the health benefits of physical activity. Many people think they are not fit enough to go regularly to a gym. The U.S. Surgeon General recommends 30 minutes of brisk walking or other similar activity on most days (4 or 5 out of 7) to reduce the risk of heart disease, diabetes, obesity, and osteoporosis. For children, experts recommend 60 minutes of exercise. Some recommend 60 minutes of moderate exercise to prevent heart disease. I believe that varied exercise routines keep it interesting and less boring. Whether you simply want to walk up and down stairs or park at the far end of a parking lot and walk—*just do it*!

Q. I am a 50-year-old male. I consider myself to be healthy. What about alcohol? What are your feelings about alcohol consumption?

A. You can read studies suggesting that red wine protects against heart disease, yet there are individuals who are allergic to the additives or the sediment in the various wines. I recommend no alcohol for those patients who want to lose weight because alcohol is a sugar, which will prevent weight loss on any dietary plan. Drinking makes your waistline bigger and increases your chance of developing blood sugar–related imbalances. The U.S. dietary guidelines state, "If you drink, do so in moderation." What does *moderation* mean? For a female, that is less than one drink and for men less than two drinks per week. Excessive alcohol consumption can lead to a dilated heart, which is a cardiomyopathy. Also, alcohol has the potential for psychological abuse and addiction. We know that pregnant women should consume no alcohol. It raises the risk of breast cancer for women. There are far more risks to drinking alcohol than there are benefits.

Q. My 23-year-old son has been experiencing frequent tightening above his heart. It does not seem to matter if he is engaged in physical activity or sitting quietly. Could this be anything that we should be alarmed about?

A. The likelihood of a 23-year-old experiencing chest tightening due to coronary artery disease is low. There are few instances in which a congenital heart disease, probably involving one of the coronary arteries, can cause chest tightening. Another congenital abnormality, called *hypertrophic cardiomyopathy* can cause chest tightening; it was previously called *idiopathic subaortic stenosis*. Much information can be found about this subject, especially whenever an article appears in the news describing how an athlete died suddenly. This congenital condition is a thickening of one of the heart's walls, which thus blocks blood flow out of the heart to the whole body. A simple echocardiogram can make this diagnosis.

Chest tightening in a young male can be due to a musculoskeletal disease. There is a documented problem called *Tietze's syndrome.* Swelling and redness on the front of the chest are rare, whereas sharp localized tenderness is common. Pressure on the cartilage near the sternum, or breastbone, and on the pectoral muscles of the chest is an essential part of a physician's examination. There are sometimes changes seen on the electrocardiogram. Emotional disorders are also common causes of chest pain. This pain is intermittent and does have to occur with exertion.

Section III. Addressing Specific Cardiac Conditions with Integrative Approaches

Q. Are most cardiac arrests due to heart disease or genetics? What are the percentages, or is everyone at risk, even without any risk factors?

A. Cardiac arrest, also known as *sudden cardiac death,* accounts for more than 400,000 deaths each year in the United States. More than 55% of these deaths are unexpected. The definition of *cardiac arrest* is an abrupt cessation of cardiac pump function. This can be reversible in a small number of cases by prompt intervention, but without it, will lead to death. The list of causes of cardiac arrest are numerous. The most common is coronary atherosclerosis. Other causes are severe heart-valve disease, especially aortic stenosis; severe cardiomyopathy with a decreased pump function; and arrhythmia.

Studies have shown that 50% of sudden cardiac death patients saw a physician one month before the event with complaints other than heart related. The ability to resuscitate a patient undergoing sudden cardiac attack is determined by the cause of the event, where it occurs, and whether there is immediate attention, such as from CPR and/or a defibrillator.

Most cardiac arrests are due to a heart problem as outlined above. There is a role that genetics plays, especially in the case of an undiagnosed congenital heart disease, such as a familial hypertrophic cardiomyopathy.

Q. I have had two bypass surgeries, two years apart. I also have a defibrillator. What vitamins or herbs would you recommend to prevent another bypass?

A. One operation is enough and two is unbelievable. I question why you needed two bypass surgeries. Did your doctor look at the other risk factors for heart diseases as he managed your lipid levels and your blood pressure? Additional risk factors that should be evaluated include levels of homocysteine, fibrinogen, cardiac C-reactive protein, and lipoprotein(a). Each of these risk factors is conventionally tested during a normal blood test analysis, and most of them if not all can be reduced with vitamins and herbs. This will decrease your risk for further surgeries and invasive testing. If you do have an abnormal stress test after your second bypass operation, I would recommend a 35-day course of EECP®. In addition, an intravenous course of chelation (EDTA) or Plaquex® (phosphatidylcholine) would be recommended.

A mechanical device, the defibrillator, for preventing sudden death was also placed. It was possibly placed if you had an abnormal arrhythmia called *ventricular tachycardia*. Individuals with two bypass operations are likely to develop a low pump function (the ejection fraction). Defibrillators are now used to prevent sudden death arrhythmias in such patients.

Vitamins and herbs recommended for preventing another bypass are numerous. It does depend on the conventional medications you are currently on.

Q. I am 57 years old and have COPD (chronic obstructive pulmonary disease). I need to know how I can better protect my heart.

A. Chronic obstructive pulmonary disease, or emphysema, is defined as abnormal enlargement or destruction of the air sacs where oxygen exchange takes place. Chronic obstructive pulmonary disease is usually preceded by years of bronchitis.

Everyday our airways are assaulted by environmental toxins we breathe in. This is especially evident in individuals who lack antioxidants in their diet and lack of additional vitamin supplementation. The key role is to prevent or decrease inflammation of the bronchial airways. Cessation of smoking is essential because it is directly correlated with the progression of COPD. Cigarette smoking is also linked to lung cancers as well as other cancers.

Vitamins and herbs can be used to prevent the development of lung disorders. The most important daily supplements for already diagnosed COPD include the essential fatty acids, 3,000–8,000 mg; magnesium

1,000–2,000 mg; vitamin C, 3,000–6,000 mg; methylsulfonylmethane (MSM) 3,000–6,000 mg; grape seed extract, 200–300 mg; bioflavonoids, such as quercetin, 2,000–3,000 mg; and N-acetyl cysteine, 500–1,500 mg. Three herbs have also been used: aloe vera (in gel form), 2–3 tablespoons/day, and extracts of *Coleus forskohlii* and *Astragalus*.

Q. How does eating sugary foods and being overweight impact the risk for heart disease?

A. The ingestion of "sugary foods," also known as the *bad carbohydrates,* increases your risk for developing diabetes. I consider diabetes in any one of its stages to be the sister disease to heart disease. Diabetes is a risk factor for cardiovascular disease. We tend to think of persons with diabetes as either on insulin or not. I would prefer to classify diabetics into four stages based on the results of a 5-hour glucose tolerance test with fasting, 1-hour and 2-hour insulin levels. Those patients with a decrease in blood sugar levels 3 to 4 hours after ingesting the glucose (sugar) drink are designated as having unstable blood sugar. This term has been loosely described as hypoglycemia. This is Stage 1.

For patients who in addition to the above also exhibit high insulin levels at the 1-hour and 2-hour marks after ingesting the glucose drink are termed *insulin resistant*. This is Stage 2. This stage is important because without starting a lifestyle dietary change and the use of certain supplements you may develop diabetes in either Stage 3 without insulin (called *diabetes Type II*) or stage 4 with insulin (called *diabetes Type I*). Type II is more common and is characterized by elevated blood sugars owing to the body's inability to use insulin correctly (insulin resistance).

More than 50% of Americans have some characteristic of one of these types. Nutritional therapy can keep the blood sugar within normal ranges by helping the body to metabolize sugar more efficiently. Some of the minerals most important in maintaining balanced sugar levels include chromium, vanadium, and manganese. Alpha lipoic acid is also used to maintain well-balanced sugar levels.

There are three herbs that I use extensively for maintaining a sugar balance. These include fenugreek, rosemary, and gymnema. In addition to gymnema's use in treating diabetes, it also has been used to treat malaria and even can aid as a laxative.

Q. What can you tell me about emu oil? I have heard that it can be beneficial for heart disease?

A. For centuries, it has been known that both the meat and oil from the emu possesses properties that are beneficial. As you know, the emu can be found roaming in Australia. Emu farms are now found in the United States. The emu oil from the fat of the bird naturally contains linolenic acid (omega-3) and linoleic acid (omega-6). The benefits of these oils in the treatment of cardiovascular diseases is outstanding. Oils are also used for their antiinflammatory and antioxidant properties. The meat itself is now used by some chefs. It is a red meat low in fat and cholesterol, yet high in protein and iron. Check the Internet for high-quality emu products.

Q. I am a patient with coronary artery disease. I have two stents. I also have high blood pressure and elevated cholesterol. I have recently started a product called Nattokinase®. What can you tell me about Nattokinase and its effects?

A. Natto is a traditional Japanese fermented soybean. Nattokinase in simple terms is an enzyme extracted from natto. It has been shown to be nutritionally supportive for the maintenance of dissolving plaque. It does this through the fibrin clotting system by breaking down the clots. Increased stickiness of platelets is involved in the development of coronary artery disease. Since many heart patients are on a blood thinner, such as Coumadin®, it is imperative that a patient be aware of the amount of vitamin K in each supplement that he or she consumes.

Vitamin K can interfere with the blood-thinning effect of Coumadin. Nattokinase, sold as Nattozyme®, does not contain vitamin K, so it will not interfere with Coumadin and other anticlotting conventional medications. However, it should be used with caution in patients on Coumadin or other anticlotting conventional medications.

Q. I have a carotid artery that is severely blocked. Are there any options other than surgery?

A. Disease of the carotid arteries (which supply blood to the head, neck, and brain), chiefly atherosclerosis, is a major health care burden. Stroke is a leading cause of death in the United States and the leading cause of long-term disability. In 1998, more than 700,000 individuals in the United States had strokes, and more than 15% of them were fatal. Currently, there are more than 3.5 million stroke survivors in the United States. Clots from the internal carotid arteries account for 40% of all cerebral strokes. We have seen several important advances in the diagnosis and treatment of the carotid arteries, which include magnetic resonance angiography and ultrasonography. These two procedures are used for the diagnosis of carotid disease and angioplasty and stents are used for the treatment of carotid disease.

We do know that stroke occurrence is generally 30 to 40% higher in men than women for ages under the age of 65 years old. We also know from statistics that there are higher mortality rates and a higher incidence of intracranial (brain) disease in people of Japanese and Chinese origin. African-American individuals constitute 20% of the patients with cerebrovascular events. Upon physical examination, the carotid arteries should be listened to with a stethoscope by the doctor. If a severe stenosis is present, the sound the physician will hear is called a *bruit*. However, note that 3 to 5% of the general population who are more than 45 years of age have a bruit without symptoms. The incidence of a carotid bruit increases with age. The treatable risk factors for the development of atherosclerosis include hypertension, diabetes, cigarette smoking, lipid levels, and alcohol consumption.

The diagnosis of carotid disease is usually made with ultrasound or angiography of the arteries. For a patient to be considered for carotid surgery (called *endarterectomy*) the amount of stenosis is usually greater than 90%. The number of carotid endarterectomies has increased in the last five years. The incidence of complications during the surgery and after the surgery still remain an issue.

The number one complication after surgery is the possibility of a stroke. There is an alternative for patients who do not want to undergo surgery or for patients with severe illnesses; it is chelation therapy. The decision to have surgery is not an easy matter when the doctor has stated, "Without this surgery you will have a stroke or heart attack." Your instant reaction is fear and panic, so, typically, you schedule the surgery. No matter how strong you feel about other treatments other than surgery, it is hard to convince your doctor about alternatives. When you ask him or her about chelation therapy, there are usually two common responses from conventional physicians. The first response is that he or she has never heard of chelation therapy. The second response is that it doesn't work and is considered nonsense. I would suggest that you refer the physician to two books that can educate him or her on EDTA chelation therapy. One is *Bypassing Bypass Surgery* and the other is *Textbook on EDTA Chelation Therapy*, second edition. Both books are written by Elmer Cranton, MD, a graduate of Harvard Medical School.

Q. How long after receiving a stent should you be taking Plavix®?

A. The usual dose of Plavix is 75 mg. The number of months a patient will be on Plavix is based on the individual. Depending on the number of stents placed and the severity of the disease, some physicians might recommend 3 to 6 months and even longer. There are some patients who have remained on Plavix.

Q. I have been told that I will be on Coumadin® for the rest of my life and I am confused about what diet to follow. I was told that vitamin K is very dangerous for me. What vegetables should I eat, and what vitamins should I avoid?

A. Avoid dark-green leafy vegetables, such as kale, Swiss chard, and spinach. Cruciferous vegetables such as broccoli and Brussels sprouts are also fairly high in vitamin K, so consume those very infrequently. Lettuce and cabbage could be consumed. In addition, you could eat asparagus, avocados, cucumbers, peppers, celery, and tomatoes. Fruits such as blueberries and grapes would be acceptable to consume in moderation. Eggs and oatmeal are acceptable breakfast options for you as well. Eat beans, nuts, and seeds—all allowable foods for someone on Coumadin.

Hyperlipidemia

Many persons living in the United States are fixated on our total cholesterol and bad cholesterol, the low-density lipoprotein (LDL). Despite evidence to the contrary, cholesterol remains and is regarded by many to be the cause of cardiovascular disease. In the 1920s when the consumption of animal fat and cholesterol was at its highest, there was little or no coronary artery disease. It wasn't until the introduction of refined carbohydrates and *trans*-fatty acids that heart disease began to emerge. Our own food pyramid and the consumption of carbohydrates has caused two epidemics, obesity and diabetes. Both are risk factors for the development of cardiovascular disease in this country.

Lowering the total cholesterol and the LDL does not always help. This has been demonstrated by the Multiple Risk Factor Intervention Trial (MRFIT), which revealed that 41% of men who died of heart attacks had total cholesterol levels less than 220. There are other studies to demonstrate that only 46% of patients who have LDL less than 160 will develop heart disease. Yet we continue to have physicians who are aggressive simply with lipid management. Prior to the latest publications, the goal LDL was less than 100. New studies are dictating an LDL less than 70. This should only be done in high-risk patients. Are these studies being funded by the manufacturers of lipid-lowering drugs? Are physicians missing the point? I do believe that lowering the total and bad cholesterol will save lives. Yet do we need pharmaceutical conventional drug therapy to achieve this goal? I think not!

Today we need to take a closer look at the LDL subtypes. There are studies now to demonstrate that particle size plays a critical role in the development of coronary artery disease and that certain diets respond to specific subtypes better than "one diet for all." The effect of lowering one's LDL particle size can be harmful if the correct dietary management is not implemented at the same time.

There are studies such as the MARS study that discuss the relationship of LDL particles and the types of atherosclerotic lesions that will develop. The management of hyperlipidemia in regards to subtypes has been well outlined in *Before the Heart Attack,* by Robert Superko, MD. This book discusses different nutritional approaches, exercise, medicine, and supplement prescriptions for various types of hyperlipidemia results.

Although statin drugs are widely prescribed in the United States, we need to discuss other ways to decrease your cholesterol and LDL. We need to steer away from the myth that cholesterol is the only risk factor for heart disease. I focus on other risk factors, which I term Longevity Risk Factors™, and include lipoprotein(a), fibrinogen, homocysteine, and high-sensitivity C-reactive protein. In 1999, a study indicated that if your triglycerides levels are greater than 138 mg/dL, you have a 16 times greater risk of having a heart attack. Therefore, we need to be aggressive in not only lowering your total and bad cholesterol, but also lowering your triglyceride level, which will then increase your good cholesterol, the high-density lipoprotein (HDL).

If we consistently bring these Longevity Risk Factors™ under control with dietary and nutritional therapies, we can live a healthier lifestyle. I get impressive results in reduction of lipid panels by eliminating sugars from the diet and restricting saturated fats. In addition, the use of pantethine, policosanol, red rice yeast, flax seed oil, green tea, and niacin can reduce your lipid profile.

The following section will discuss answers to your commonly asked questions regarding your high lipid levels.

You're on the Air...
Q. Are there vitamins I should be taking to lower my cholesterol?

A. We are a society fixated on total cholesterol and the bad cholesterol, LDL. Although these are important risk factors, we also need to consider lowering your triglyceride level and increasing your good cholesterol. There is a complex of vitamins that lower your cholesterol. These include policosanol, gugulipids (although recent reports are controversial) pantethine, and lecithin. There are studies to validate a reduction in total cholesterol and your bad cholesterol using both green and black teas.

In today's society, most individuals with high cholesterol are prescribed a statin drug. Statin drugs do deplete an essential vita-nutrient, coenzyme Q_{10}. The side effects of the statins are well documented and include an elevation of liver enzymes as well as muscle aches (myalgias).

Q. Is there a non-drug treatment for small, dense LDL? Do you recommend screening for small, dense LDL?

A. Great strides have been made in the testing for LDL. The size does make the difference. If you have a large amount of the small, dense LDL, you have been classified as a Pattern B type. On the other end of the spectrum, if your LDL are predominantly large, you are classified as Pattern A. Small LDL (Pattern B) carries an increased risk for cardiovascular events and development of diabetes. Studies do indicate that Pattern B patients have the most rapid progression of coronary artery disease, yet you need to understand that it is the most treatable following dietary restrictions and supplement use. Most individuals with Pattern B also exhibit a high triglyceride level and thus will have a low HDL level (the good cholesterol). This is reversible. First, you follow a low-carbohydrate lifestyle by eliminating the simple, refined ones. This includes pastas, breads, certain fruits, and, of course, sugar. We also use a diet that is low in saturated fat. This does mean less intake of red meats. You should concentrate on lean meats, such as chicken, turkey, and fish. Be aware of certain fish, such as tuna and swordfish, as they contain higher levels of mercury. Second, exercise is an important step. Find an exercise you can enjoy—whether walking, hiking, bicycle riding, or swimming. Incorporate this exercise into your daily routine. In addition, certain supplements, such as niacin, should be added to the regimen.

Q. How effective is niacin in lowering cholesterol levels?

A. Niacin is extremely effective in lowering cholesterol. Studies show that niacin can lower the bad cholesterol, LDL, by up to 25%. In addition, niacin decreases the triglyceride levels and increases your good cholesterol, HDL. Niacin also can decrease the independent cardiovascular risk factor lipoprotein(a).

Niacin should not be taken in high doses to lower cholesterol without consideration of how this will impact the other B vitamins in your body. The B vitamins are meant to be taken together, so when using niacin to lower cholesterol, it is necessary to take a B-complex vitamin as well to ensure that the other B's don't get depleted or offset by the niacin.

Because of its vasodilating properties, within minutes of taking niacin patients experience a skin flushing that often appears as redness and swelling on areas of the body; the sensation is accompanied by heat and often itchiness. This lasts for about 10 minutes and subsides, but is often uncomfortable for the patient. To minimize the flushing, take niacin with food, or cut the tablet in half and take smaller doses throughout the day rather than one big dose. Niacin is also available in a timed-release form, and this too can minimize flushing.

Q. How can I decrease the risk of high LDL cholesterol?

A. The best way to decrease your risk of an elevated LDL would be to cut back on certain fats in your diet, and to completely avoid fried foods and heavy sauces like those found in some Chinese foods. Omit bacon, sausage, and other fatty foods from your diet, substituting them with turkey bacon or tofu sausage. Eat lean cuts of beef, such as filet mignon, no more than once a week and monitor the amount and types of cheese you eat. It is best that you choose the leaner cheeses such as goat and feta cheese and to use those in moderation. Try to obtain your fats from plant sources such as walnuts, almonds, and avocado.

As mentioned in the previous question, niacin would also be a wonderful supplement to include if you're concerned about an elevated

LDL. Be sure, however, to take it in combination with the other B vitamins.

Q. My 12-year-old son is 52 pounds overweight, and recent blood tests showed that he had high triglyceride levels. What does this mean, and how can I lower his triglycerides?

A. Obesity and Diabetes are two epidemics this country now faces. With more than 50% of overweight Americans, it was only a matter of time before the epidemic trickled over into the pediatric population. Childhood obesity is a major health concern. I am concerned that your child has a high triglyceride level. A careful family history should be taken to see if any member of the family also has a problem with triglycerides. Has diabetes ever been discussed? I would recommend a 5-hour glucose tolerance test with insulin levels for your son. High triglyceride levels are the most common in metabolic syndromes, such as diabetes, which is now recognized as an independent risk factor for coronary artery disease.

A major goal for children and adolescents is in the maintenance of normal growth and development. A complete nutritional assessment for your child, including food history, biochemical interactions, assessment of family concerns, and social issues, should be done. It has been shown that the best way to lower triglycerides is by decreasing the intake of refined carbohydrates, and to start an exercise regimen. I do realize that meal planning for a child is difficult especially when school lunch programs are so high in refined carbohydrates. The fact that he is overweight would also be a good indication that he consumes high amounts of sugars and refined carbohydrates.

The first thing to do is change his diet. This is more challenging to do with children because they don't yet understand the concept of illness. Because of this, there is no great motivation to eat healthfully, because at their age, health is taken for granted. I would start out by removing all junk food from the home. This would include candy, soda, chips, cookies, and ice cream. Simply never keep it in the home to lessen temptation.

Switch from white bread to a hearty seven-grain or sprouted bread. Give your child a healthy breakfast that includes a couple of eggs for protein and a piece of good toast. Send your child off to school with a banana and some nuts for a snack. Offer nutritious dinners that include lean protein like fish or chicken. To get your child to eat vegetables, combine a package of broccoli and cheese with a package of plain broccoli; in this way, you dilute the amount of cheese, yet provide a sufficient amount to enhance flavor.

Other suggestions would be to

- change from drinking whole milk to 1%.
- dilute fruit juices with water.
- encourage exercise.
- participate in yoga for children.
- participate in school sports.
- encourage walking.
- enroll your child in karate or tae kwon do. These would be a good source of exercise, and exercise has shown to lower triglycerides.

Q. Can taking vitamins and supplements help to lower a fairly active 58-year-old male's triglyceride blood levels? High triglycerides are an important indictor for the development of coronary artery disease and type II diabetes.

A. The best way to lower your triglycerides is diet and exercise. However, niacin can be used. Mainstream medicine does consider niacin to be a drug and it is now available by conventional prescription. A comfortable dose can be from 100 to 500 mg with an increasing dose as tolerated. I say as tolerated because niacin can cause a flush. The flush is quite harmless and wears off when niacin is taken on a regular basis. The development of a vitamin, inositol hexanicotinate, was developed to gain the effects of niacin without the side effect liabilities.

Section III. Addressing Specific Cardiac Conditions with Integrative Approaches

Arrhythmias

Arrhythmia is a common medical term for an abnormal heart rhythm. Other terms that patients use are palpitations, skipped beats, extra beats, and pounding in the chest. If these extra beats persist, an arrhythmia can occur. The most common is called *atrial fibrillation*. It is important that a patient can detect and palpate his or her own pulse. The best pulse to check is the radial pulse: the radial artery is located on the thumb side of the underside of the wrist. The important three questions a patient can ask themselves while palpating their own radial pulse are (1) is the pulse regular or irregular, (2) is the pulse fast or slow, and (3) are they symptomatic with shortness of breath or dizziness or not.

For example, a pulse that is totally irregular and fast, with or without symptoms, signifies atrial fibrillation. Since atrial fibrillation in patients older than 65 years carries an increased risk for stroke, it is important to discuss this arrhythmia.

Causes of atrial fibrillation are

- presence of heart-valve disease

- coronary artery disease

- abnormal thyroid function

There are patients who have a no significant valve disease, nonobstructive coronary artery disease, and a normal thyroid panel who still have atrial fibrillation. These patients are placed on a conventional antiarrhythmic drug and even warfarin (Coumadin®, a blood thinner) with no known cause of why they have atrial fibrillation.

There are nonconventional causes for atrial fibrillation, such as unstable blood sugar, allergies, infections, and even heavy metal toxicity. There is a role for some antiarrhythmic drugs for decreasing heart rates and even converting rhythms to normal. However, as with any medication, there are significant side effects. These side effects deter patients from either starting the drug or even changing from one class of antiarrhythmic to another class. Some patients even steer away from doctors who prescribe these medications.

There are also vitamins and herbs that can prevent arrhythmias and some can slow the heart rate better than prescribed medications. Some of these herbs include hawthorn, motherwort, and night blooming cactus. Some of the vitamins that are used include magnesium, calcium, and potassium. Since there are no regulatory bodies governing the use of vitamins and herbs, it is imperative that a patient discuss any supplement or over-the-counter herbs with their doctors. There are many drug–vitamin and drug–herb interactions.

This section will not only educate you on the use of vitamins and herbs, but will also answer your commonly asked questions.

You're on the Air…
Q. What vitamins or supplements would you recommend to treat an irregular heartbeat?

A. An irregular heartbeat, or a palpitation, is a common reason why a patient seeks medical attention. These extra single beats can occur rapidly or together. This is now called an *arrhythmia*. For simplicity and educational purposes, you need to answer three basic questions first. Are the palpitations (1) irregular or regular; (2) fast or slow; and (3) with or without other symptoms, such as shortness of breath, fainting, or even chest pain. This information during the medical history is important for the physician. A simple 24-hour ECG tracing or Holter monitor can make this differential quickly. There are three conventional cardiological causes for an arrhythmia.

1. Heart disease involving a leaky (regurgitant) or tight (stenotic) valve can cause palpitations. An ultrasound of the heart (echocardiogram) can diagnose these conditions.

2. Coronary artery disease, partial or complete blockage of a coronary artery, can cause palpitations. A stress test can diagnose this condition.

3. The third cause of palpitations can be an overactive thyroid. A simple blood test can diagnose this.

There are other nonconventional causes of palpitations that can be discussed. An unstable blood sugar is an important cause of palpitations and frequently not considered. When a patient comes to me for a consultation regarding palpitations, an extensive food history is asked. For example, in many cases an episode of palpitations was preceded by an intake of a carbohydrate three hours earlier. After ingesting a carbohydrate (pasta, bread, cake, etc.) there is an elevation in the blood sugars. If the patient has an unstable blood sugar, the blood sugar levels will decrease three to four hours later.

The way our body compensates for a low blood sugar is to release adrenaline from the adrenal glands, which are situated on top of the kidneys. The increase in adrenaline increases the heart rate, thus causing palpitations. A change in dietary lifestyle can be life saving. Another important cause of palpitations is allergies. Most consider an allergic reaction to exhibit in the form of rash or itching. Certain foods and chemicals can cause palpitations in a majority of patients. Extensive food and environmental allergy testing should be considered. One area that is underexamined is the role of mercury and heavy metal toxicity causing palpitations.

The public awareness of the possible dangers of amalgam fillings (which 50% contain mercury) began with Dr. Hal Huggins. As early as the 17th century, mad hatter's disease was recognized as exposure to mercury vapors in the hat making industry in Europe. This was due to the neurotoxic effects of mercury. The effects of mercury go beyond the neurotoxic effect. Symptoms of mercury toxicity include fatigue, tremors, bad taste in mouth, joint pain, headache, dizziness, ringing in the ears, and arrhythmias. When a patient presents with atrial fibrillation, a provocative challenge test for heavy metals should be done.

Mercury is an irritant to the cardiac electrical system. In 1999, an article was published in a well-known cardiology journal discussing the toxic level of mercury found in heart muscle in patients with a dilated heart (a cardiomyopathy). I do recommend that patients consider removing their amalgams. When the amalgams are removed, a chelating agent should be given, such as dimercapto-propane sulfonate (DMPS) and vitamin C intravenously. There are many vitamin and herbs that can be used to treat irregular heart beat. Some of the most important minerals include magnesium, manganese, potassium and chromium.

There are multiple herbs in tincture form that I recommend for arrhythmias. These include Hawthorne, Scotch broom, night blooming cactus, motherwort, and lily of the valley. These herbs are often described as heart tonics. The herb foxglove (digitalis) is left out here even though it is used by conventional cardiologists for the treatment of congestive heart failure. Lily of the valley was used as a celestial potion in combination with other herbs to conserve youth and to cure impotence. The fruits and seeds of the lily of the valley are toxic if eaten. This is a reason why when planted in a vegetable garden no animals disturb your tomatoes, carrots, and lettuce. There are drug–herbal interactions with all of these herbs in a patient who is also taking the conventional medications beta-blockers (e.g., atenolol), cardiac glycosides (e.g., digoxin) and calcium channel blockers (e.g., verapamil and cardizem).

Q. My son is 20-years-old and has been experiencing arrhythmic events for several years. All of his tests have been done, but no medication has been prescribed for him. These episodes are scary for both him and us. Can you recommend

Section III. Addressing Specific Cardiac Conditions with Integrative Approaches

vitamins or other nutritional strategies to help minimize these episodes?

A. First of all, what kind of arrhythmia has been diagnosed in your 20-year-old son? The most common arrhythmia in his age group is supraventricular tachycardia. This arrhythmia originates from the AV node within the heart and is considered an accessory pathway. Today with the advancement of nonsurgical ablation for these arrhythmias, many patients do not require medication. This arrhythmia sometimes occurs in association with another problem called *Wolff-Parkinson-White* syndrome.

Attacks of this intermittent tachycardia are usually easily converted to normal rhythm by drugs or certain procedures to increase vagal tones. These vagal tone procedures include bearing down, as when having a bowel motion, blowing into a balloon, or the use of an ice collar or dunking the individual's head in a bowl of ice. There are many drugs used to prevent recurrent episodes, such as digitalis, quinidine, procainamide, beta-blockers, and flecainide. All of these drugs have side effects and I would probably not recommend them to a 20-year-old without further work-up.

If your son had all normal invasive testing including an electrophysiological study to determine the type of arrhythmia, then I would search for a nonconventional cause of his palpitations. These would include a provocative challenge test for heavy metals, an allergy panel, a glucose tolerance test as outlined in this book, and an infectious work-up.

Q. I was diagnosed with atrial fibrillation at age 50. I am now age 58. I do not have any symptoms, and have intermittent atrial fibrillation. I am taking 5 mg of Coumadin® and a

drug called sotalol. I have been tested with various tests and everything I am told is normal. Do I need to take these drugs?

A. As you stated, you have had all conventional cardiac testing. There are other nonconventional causes for atrial fibrillation. I would search for the cause of your atrial fibrillation. I would recommend a 6-hour provocative urine toxicology challenge for heavy metals, especially mercury. Mercury is cardiotoxic to the electrical system. If elevated, it can be decreased with chelators, thus causing fewer episodes of intermittent atrial fibrillation. Another cause of atrial fibrillation is infection. I would recommend the conventional blood test cardiac C-reactive protein. If elevated I would search for 20 or more infections that can contribute to atrial fibrillation. I would recommend IgG and IgM antibody testing. In addition, potassium and magnesium have been used for controlling arrhythmias.

Q. I am overweight and sometimes feel flutters in my chest. Do you feel that this is related?

A. It would be wise for you to have your glucose levels checked. Fluttering could be a sign of hypoglycemia, or an imbalanced blood sugar. The fact that you are overweight suggests this to be the case. Do you crave sugar? Do you consume a lot of refined carbohydrates like bread, pasta, and potatoes? These are signs that may point toward hypoglycemia. When you eat sugar, your glucose levels shoot up, only to drop down precipitously, often causing palpitations, or flutters. Therefore, I would suggest a 5-hour glucose tolerance test with insulin levels. Other nonconventional causes of "flutters" to pursue after doing the conventional cardiac testing would be mercury toxicity, allergy work-up, and infectious work-up. It would also be useful to wear an event monitor that has a button you can push whenever you feel these flutters. This would allow the physician to determine the type of irregularity you are experiencing. This can allow him to detect if these flutters are being generated from the top chambers of the heart, the atria, or the bottom chambers of the heart, the ventricles.

Q. My cardiologist says there is nothing I can do for the calcium on the main artery and the blockage is 55%.

A. *There is something you can do.* Mainstream cardiologists treat symptoms and, observe and perform tests every year until the blockage becomes greater than 70%. When the blockage is greater than 70%, it is possible that your stress test will be abnormal. An initial evaluation will determine if you are a candidate for EECP® (enhanced external counterpulsation). In addition, you need to start a prevention program so as to not allow the natural history of calcium blockages to build up. This can include chelation or Plaquex®, both of which are described in this book.

Q. I am a twenty-three-year-old female that has been diagnosed with multiple sclerosis (MS) and have been recently diagnosed with supraventricular tachycardia. Is it possible that MS created the heart problem? What supplements would you recommend for these conditions?

A. Multiple sclerosis and the arrhythmia supraventricular tachycardia are two different conditions. We do know that with multiple sclerosis the body mistakenly identifies and destroys the protective sheath of all nerves. Some postulate that infections can contribute to MS, and another cause that I can relate to the arrhythmias is the accumulation of high levels of toxic metals, such as mercury. The body's own immune system will consider this mercury laden in the brain to be foreign and it will begin to destroy it.

Mercury is also toxic to the electrical system of the heart and can cause arrhythmia. I have seen excessive metal load as mercury to be associated with atrial fibrillation, which is another atrial rhythm like supraventricular tachycardia. Since we are discussing these two independent diseases, I would recommend a provocation challenge heavy metal test and to proceed based on these results. The most common cause of toxic mercury levels in the body might lie in your dental amalgam fillings, which are made up of greater than 50% mercury. When I was the chief of medicine at the Atkins Center in New York City, Dr. Robert C. Atkins and I treated MS with intravenous calcium amino ethanol phosphate (AEP), with one vial every two days.

Currently there are no proven treatments for changing or reversing the course of MS and preventing further attacks. The medical nutritional therapy in my view is extensive and many diets have been tried, the most common diet that has been used is a low-fat and gluten free one. There are others, such as pectin-free and allergen-free diets that have been used. Yet there are no valid clinical trials supporting the efficacy of nutrition in delaying progression. I do not think this means that diets and supplements do not work. I believe they have beneficial results in some patients. The additional benefits of safflower and soybean oil have produced some benefits. Other studies have used eicosapentaenoic (EPA) and docosahexaenoic (DHA) oils at doses at an average of 1.5 grams. I have used these oils in much higher doses, with an average dose of 3.0 grams. Other supplements that I use include octacosanol, sphingomyelin, pancreatic enzymes, and high-dose folic acid.

Q. Are there adrenal supplements that can help with anxiety-related premature ventricular contractions, or "extra beats," or other arrhythmias aggravated by elevated cortisol and/or irregular cortisol swings?

A. Arrhythmias are discussed elsewhere in this book so allow me to address anxiety at this point. There are many herbs and supplements that help with anxiety. Living life on life's terms creates anxiety in this most stressful environment. Anxiety can be alleviated or decreased by changing your dietary lifestyle and incorporating other techniques such as exercise, energy medicine, guided imagery, and yoga, into your life.

The vitamin and mineral supplements that have been used for anxiety are magnesium, inositol, calcium, and the B vitamins. There are herbs that have also been used. Valerian has been used to treat restlessness, insomnia, and anxiety. The primary effect of St. John's wort is acting on the serotonin receptor sites, creating a feeling of calmness. For this reason, caution should be used when taking any of these herbs in combination with prescription serotonin drugs such as Celexa®, Paxil®, and Zoloft®. Kava has been used as an antianxiety drug. There are many known interactions of kava with prescription drugs. The sedative action of kava is unlike any other. It acts directly on the parts of the brain that generate emotion and motivation. Although there have been reports of the use of skullcap for anxiety, its primary use has been to treat seizure and spastic disorders. Passion flower is used as a sedative and to treat anxiety like the herb motherwort.

The hormonal influences on anxiety are well known. Most of the studies have been with an overactive thyroid (hyperthyroidism, Hashimoto's thyroiditis). Nevertheless, there needs to be a balance of other hormones, especially of the adrenal gland, primarily involving cortisol function.

Phosphatidyl serine has been shown to decrease cortisol levels, thereby relieving stress and anxiety. The dose for this would be 600 mg daily in divided doses.

Valvular Heart Disease, Cardiomyopathy, and Congestive Heart Failure

Valvular heart disease is a group of conditions that can lead to congestive heart failure. Congestive heart failure (CHF) affects 5 million Americans every year. There are many conventional studies, with the acronyms ELITE, CHARM, and Val-HEFT, that demonstrate the benefits of conventional medications in treating heart failure.

To understand valvular heart disease, you need to understand some basic heart anatomy. There are four heart valves: two valves that separate the top chambers (the atria) from the bottom chambers (the ventricles). Thus, these are called *atrioventricular valves*. The mitral valve separates the left atrium from the left ventricle, and the tricuspid valve separates the right atrium from the right ventricle. There are also two valves that separate the ventricles from the body. The aortic valve separates the left ventricle from the body on the left and the pulmonic valve separates the right ventricle from the lungs on the right. These are called semilunar valves. Any of these valves can leak (can be regurgitant or insufficient) or can be tight (stenotic). There are some patients born with valve conditions. Some patients acquire valve disease by such causes as rheumatic fever, heart attacks, and infections (endocarditis). The natural history of valve disease is that they progress. Symptoms of valvular heart disease include shortness of breath, palpitations (arrhythmias), dizziness, and even chest pain.

I am not opposed to valve surgery for replacing a damaged valve. I use the analogy of a song that I listened to as a teenager. Kay Kyser had a #1 hit song called "On a Slow Boat to China." A patient who has a valve condition, if left untreated, will end up in China sooner than those patients who choose to slow the trip, or the progression of the disease. With the use of conventional medications such as diuretics, ACE (angiotensin-converting enzyme) inhibitors or ARB (angiotensin-receptor-blocking) medications and certain herbs and vitamins, the progression of valvular disease is slower. The practice of integrating conventional medicines and herbs is to help relieve the patient of symptoms. I see many patients for a second opinion, especially those who do not want to have surgery. By taking a careful history and physical to determine whether the patient is symptomatic and by implementing some amino acids, such as taurine and carnitine, the progression can be slower. There is a critical time at which surgery should be performed.

Valvular heart disease, as stated earlier, can lead to CHF. Independent of valve disease, CHF can be caused by coronary artery disease or a cardiomyopathy (dilation of the heart). A cardiomyopathy can occur with or without coronary artery disease. Those patients who have a cardiomyopathy caused by coronary artery blockage are referred to as having *ischemic* cardiomyopathy. Most patients have a cardiomyopathy without a blockage.

The most common cause of a dilated cardiomyopathy in this country is alcohol abuse. The second cause is a viral infection that affected the cardiac muscle. A newly recognized cause, previously not considered, is heavy metal toxicity. Metals such as mercury, antimony, and cadmium become deposited in the heart muscle. A cardiomyopathy whether ischemic or not will lead to a decrease in the pumping function. The normal ejection fraction is 55 to 75%. Numerous studies show the benefit for coenzyme Q_{10} and carnitine in increasing the ejection fraction of the heart.

The use of enhanced external counterpulsation (EECP) has been used for heart failure patients with Class III and Class IV American Heart Association classifications. This noninvasive and nontraumatic treatment was initially approved for its benefits in patients with coronary artery disease.

A patient entering a hospital with CHF complicated by a heart attack twenty years ago faced 80% to 90% mortality. Today, with the advancement in technology and medications, the mortality rate for the same patients is 22%.

The question is, "Can we further reduce the mortality?" The answer is, "Yes, we can with the use of lifestyle modifications, vitamin/mineral supplements, herbs, and EECP."

The next section will answer some of your most commonly asked questions.

You're on the Air...
Q. I was diagnosed with mitral valve prolapse (MVP), and my physician prescribed atenolol, which I have been taking ever since. Can you recommend ways I can improve my condition?

A. Mitral valve prolapse, also known as *floppy valve syndrome*, is a condition in which there is a displacement of any portion of the mitral valve leaflets. Other names it has been known by are *Barlow's syndrome, effort syndrome,* and *soldier's heart.* The classic mitral valve prolapse is called *myxomatous mitral valve prolapse,* or a redundancy, or thickening, in certain portions of the mitral valve. Most patients with MVP are asymptomatic, but some seek care for palpitations, atypical chest pain, and shortness of breath. If you are without symptoms from MVP, no treatment is required. I would reassure you that if you have no symptoms, a beta-blocker such as atenolol is not needed. However, if there are symptoms such as palpitations, a beta-blocker would be recommended to decrease the heart rate. I usually recommend hawthorn either in capsule form or tincture. In addition, the usage of minerals such as magnesium, potassium, and manganese will alleviate the palpitations. I have prescribed additional water intake, with a ½ teaspoon of salt in a 32-oz container. This allows more volume in the heart, thus decreasing the amount of prolapse and lessening the symptoms. This should only be done if there is no evidence of congestive heart failure or hypertension. Usually patients with MVP have a low blood pressure.

Q. Can vitamins and supplements be used to correct mild heart valve irregularities?

A. There aren't any vitamins that help correct a valve disease. Valve disease tends to progress over time. However, there are supplements that can help slow the progression and maintain a healthy strong heart. These include L-taurine, L-carnitine, coenzyme Q_{10}, and magnesium. Herbs that promote good heart function are hawthorn, ginkgo, garlic, and cayenne pepper.

The most commonly diagnosed valve condition is mitral valve regurgitation. This is due to a backflow of blood into the left atrium from the left ventricle. This condition can be acute, chronic, or even intermittent. Some of the causes of mitral valve regurgitation are mitral valve calcification, a flail (damaged) chord, infarction of the papillary muscle (which supports the chord), infection of the valve (endocarditis), and congenital problems. The earliest symptom a patient will seek medical attention for is fatigue. Other symptoms include shortness of breath, chest pain, leg swelling, and congestive heart failure. A good physical exam will detect a murmur, which can be evaluated and diagnosed by an ultrasound of the heart (echocardiogram). An electrocardiogram (ECG) is not beneficial in these patients because their ECGs can be normal or with few abnormalities.

Patients with moderate-to-severe mitral valve regurgitation do require antibiotic prophylaxis prior to dental and other medical procedures. There are numerous conventional drugs that are used to prevent symptoms, including diuretics; nitrate derivatives; ACE inhibitors, such as enalapril (Vasotec®) and ramipril (Altace®); and digoxin. Even beta-blockers are used for some patients. There is a role for conventional medications in preventing symptoms. There also is a role for taurine, carnitine, and coenzyme Q_{10} to strengthen the heart muscle. Any supplement or herb that is used should be discussed with your health care practitioners because there are well-known interactions with conventional medications.

There is a role for valvular surgery or replacement. This can be done with a metal valve or a tissue valve. A patient must understand that a metal valve requires life-long anticoagulation therapy with Coumadin®.

Q. My sister-in-law is 5 months pregnant and the baby has bicuspid atresia. Can you tell me what the life expectancy of this child might be?

A. I will assume that bicuspid atresia is the same at mitral atresia. This conclusion is because the mitral valve is a bicuspid valve, normally. There is an aortic bicuspid valve, which is a congenital abnormality; the normal aortic valve has three cusps. Bicuspid atresia was first described by Dr. Lev in 1952, where he discussed the congenital malformations characterized by a underdevelopment of components on the left side of the heart. This can include absence of the mitral valve or absence of the aortic valve. The term *mitral atresia*, with a normal aortic valve, refers to the condition in which the mitral valve is absent and there is no opening between the left atrium (top chamber) and either ventricle (the bottom chambers). The heart functions as if there is one ventricle. Symptoms can range from mild to severe. Some of these symptoms include shortness of breath, chest pain, and palpitations. If at birth this congenital disorder is severe, the baby can be blue and even have failure to thrive. With the advancements in technology in areas of congenital heart disease, we are having more infants and children reach adulthood. Children born with severe congenital heart defects in the 1950 and 1960 did not have the chance that surgery offers today.

Q. Is Coenzyme Q_{10} used in the treatment of cardiomyopathy?

A. Coenzyme Q_{10} (CoQ_{10}), or ubiquinone, was first isolated from beef heart by Fredrick Crane in 1957. Two doctors documented CoQ_{10} deficiency in human heart disease in 1972, but it was not included in mainstream conventional cardiology textbooks until 1997. What's the mystery? There is none. Multiple books and research have documented the beneficial effects of CoQ_{10}, for energy metabolism, and for its use in heart disease. I have found CoQ_{10} useful in 10 mg up to as high as 2,400 mg. The type of cardiovascular disease needs to be evaluated to determine how much CoQ_{10}. The average person should have an intake of 100 mg to 300 mg of CoQ_{10}, with higher doses to be used in congestive heart failure. Recent studies have documented the beneficial use of 1,800 to 2,400 mg in patients with Parkinson's disease, thus decreasing the progression of the disease

Q. My brother is 56-years-old and has been diagnosed with congestive heart failure. His ejection fraction was 26%, and now it is 34%. What are the causes of his heart failure and what can he do? He takes so many cardiac medications.

A. There are many causes for heart failure. The two main causes are valvular heart disease and cardiomyopathy. The most common valves that predispose to heart failure are diseases of the mitral and aortic valves.

The most common cardiomyopathy in this country is alcohol abuse. The second most common cause is a viral infection. Your brother should be considered for a heart transplant if there are no contraindications. There are multiple vitamins and herbs that can be used with his conventional medications. Of course, these vitamins and herbs can have interactions. I would suggest your brother find a practitioner that is familiar with herbs and vitamins for the heart. I would recommend high-dose CoQ_{10} and carnitine because both have had beneficial results in increasing the ejection fraction (pump function) of the heart.

Q. I am 81-years-old with a leaky aortic valve, which I have had for years. I take one 50-mg Cozaar® every day. Is there

anything I can do to improve my condition or something I should avoid to keep it from getting worse?

A. At this age with no symptoms, I doubt that your aortic insufficiency (leakage) will progress. I cannot prevent what is already there or reverse what is there. What I can do is limit its progression by suggesting certain vitamins and herbs.

Cozaar® is an ARB (angiotensin receptor blocker) drug used to treat heart failure. Other conventional drugs used for heart failure include the ACE drugs, certain beta-blockers, and diuretics. The diuretics further deplete minerals as well as thiamin, or vitamin B_1. Replenishing the body's store of thiamin is essential. Most, if not all, of the B vitamins (especially vitamin B_6) act as diuretics and prevent water retention.

There are three suggestions to help strengthen your heart, which would include taking CoQ_10, taurine, and carnitine. L-Taurine is an amino acid that regulates our minerals, keeping potassium and magnesium inside the cells and keeping the extra sodium out of the cells. This functions as a natural diuretic and works with the kidneys—not against them as conventional diuretics do. They encourage the excretion of extra body fluids, which takes the pressure off our blood vessels. Taurine also strengthens the heart muscle function and stabilizes calcium levels. I regularly use taurine in the treatment of valvular heart disease, congestive heart failure, blood pressure, and arrhythmias.

Q. Can an enlarged heart go back to normal size? I am 56 years old with a history of hypertension and a 30-year cardiac history, but no heart attacks as yet.

A. An enlarged heart is a condition termed *cardiomegaly*. The presence of cardiomegaly on a routine chest X-ray warrants the physician to determine its cause. In your case, a diagnosis of hypertension and a 30-year cardiac history is the cause. You stated that you have not had a

Section III. Addressing Specific Cardiac Conditions with Integrative Approaches

heart attack, but do you have any coronary artery disease? Do you have stents or partial blockage of any coronary artery?

Studies have demonstrated that heart size can reverse after bypass, when the pumping function of the heart muscle is restored. The use of CoQ_{10} is essential for any cardiac patient and its deficiency is seen in all untreated cardiac patients. Deficiencies of CoQ_{10} have been documented in many cardiac conditions, such as congestive heart failure, hypertension, coronary artery disease, valvular heart disease, and those following coronary artery bypass grafting.

<u>Hypertension</u>

Hypertension (high blood pressure) is the number-one chronic cardiovascular disease in America, with more than 50 million being affected every year. Hypertension is a risk factor for the development of coronary artery disease, stroke, peripheral vascular disease, and cardiac failure. It is prevalent in this country, yet overall, we do a poor job in trying to treat it.

Despite numerous studies and treatment protocols, only 33% of Americans are aware of this risk. Elevated systolic blood pressure (the first number) is the leading cardiovascular disease, and blood pressure does increase with aging. The adage that a normal blood pressure reading is 130/80 is a fallacy. By a new classification, called the *JNC 7*, 130/80 is considered pre-hypertensive. Lifestyle modification is the key: reducing alcohol, reducing caffeine, smoking cessation, dietary restriction, and exercise are crucial to the health of the heart.

There is a need for conventional pharmacological medications in the role of treating high blood pressure. I am not totally opposed to using medications, especially the newer class—angiotensin receptor blockers (ARB), such as Benecar®—and even using the older conventional types—the diuretics, such as hydrochlorothiazide. Diuretics synergize and work well with either ARB or ACE drugs. There are compelling indications for the use of other individual drug classes. For example, post–heart attack patients can benefit from the use of beta-blockers.

Yet, do we always need to use a prescription drug to lower blood pressure? It is my opinion that blood pressure can be lowered with the use of certain vitamins and herbs. You may ask, are there double-blind studies to show the efficacy of herbs and vitamins to lower blood pressure? The answer is no, yet do we need those studies when there is an overabundance of clinical patient measurements that demonstrate that herbs and vitamins do lower blood pressure? Again, the answer is no.

I want each of my patients to achieve their individual blood pressure goal. If this means the integration of a pharmaceutical medication with the use of taurine, magnesium, hawthorn, and the rest, then I have no objection. I continually see patients on three to five different blood pressure medications for blood pressure control. I always integrate herbs in these patient's protocols in an attempt to lower some of their conventional medications. I do this with close monitoring of the patient's blood pressure and always with the intention of "first, do no harm."

There are side effects with any prescribed conventional drug. Side effects are the most common reasons why patients do not want to start to take a medication. Often, they experience a side effect and want to discontinue the use of the conventional medication. After spending time with each patient, I find that they are likely to lower the dosage of a conventional medication if I add herbs or vitamins into their regimen.

The use of home blood pressure monitoring is recommended. I recommend an Omron model for most of my patients. However, I am usually careful when interpreting results. There are some patients who always consider themselves disabled and will always report higher home blood pressure readings. On the other hand, there are some patients totally resistant to conventional medications that have been prescribed and always report lower home readings.

As a cardiologist, I review literature and studies on different areas within the field of cardiology. I am concerned about microalbumin (a protein) excreted in the urine. This is a risk factor for organ damage resulting from hypertension. This test is always given to the diabetic patient; however, I screen all hypertensive patients. There is a need to decrease albuminuria through the use conventional medications to help prevent irreversible kidney damage.

The next section will focus on questions regarding commonly prescribed medications and the use of herbs and vitamins to treat high blood pressure.

You're on the Air...
Q. Are there vitamins I should be taking to lower my blood pressure?

A. There are many vitamins and herbs to help lower your blood pressure. The top two vita-nutrients that should be considered are magnesium in doses from 400–800 mg per day and CoQ_{10} in a dose of 100–300 mg per day. An important herb, hawthorn, is also beneficial.

Other important supplements include chromium, vitamin C, and vitamin E. L-Taurine and L-carnitine, two amino acids, have also been proven to be effective.

Q. My mother-in-law has high blood pressure. She was placed on Cozaar®. What are your thoughts about this medication?

A. Cozaar® is a blood pressure medication in the class of angiotensin receptor–blocking (ARB) drugs. I consider these the second generation of another class of blood pressure medications, called ACE (angiotensin-converting enzyme) inhibitors. These are the two classes of medications that I utilize in my practice. Each of these medications is effective, with minimal side effects. I monitor the use of these medications and their effectiveness by urine samples of albumin. If a patient has high blood pressure, is not on any medication, and is excreting albumin in their urine, there is a definite need for either class. As they start either of the classes, the excretion of albumin in the urine decreases. This means that the medication is working.

There are other drugs within the ARB class that I utilize more frequently, such as Benecar®. I choose my conventional medications wisely depending on the race, age, and compliance of my patients. I also read the current research on one drug in a class versus another drug in the same class. I am not inclined to use a medication based on the pharmaceutical samples that are in my office cabinets.

There are also multiple herbs and vitamins that have been used to lower blood pressure. I recommend magnesium, calcium, and potassium to lower blood pressure. L-Taurine and L-carnitine are two amino acids that have proven to be effective. Herbs such as hawthorn can also be used.

Q. How do you distinguish between the so-called white coat hypertension and "real "hypertension?

A. White coat hypertension is a well-recognized condition in which a patient's blood pressure is elevated when in a doctor's office. The increased blood pressure is due to anxiety and stress, or the fear of being in a physician's office. Blood pressure measurements should be taken in three positions: sitting, standing, and lying flat, and in both arms. Treatment for high blood pressure should not begin until after the second or third visit to the doctor's office. This general rule can be broken if the patient has complaints such as dizziness, shortness of breath, and chest pain. I also prescribe that the patient wear a home 24-hour monitor. This monitor allows the physician to view the blood pressure readings in the patient's home environment and while the patient is performing his or her daily activities. A cardiac work-up should be done, including an echocardiogram (ECG) and a stress test. Blood tests for Longevity Risk Factors™ should be done as well.

There are lifestyle modifications for reducing and controlling blood pressure. There are various techniques in stress management, such as yoga, meditation, hypnotherapy, biofeedback, and *qi-gong*. Regular exercise reduces stress and blood pressure and is highly recommended. I encourage patients to do an exercise that is fun for them. I find swimming and walking to be the most effective for the older age population. Other simple rules to follow to reduce blood pressure include

1. Reduce weight

2. Reduce intake of salt

3. Reduce or eliminate caffeinated beverages, alcohol, and smoking

4. Eat more foods high in omega-3 oils

5. Decrease saturated fat intake

6. Start a vitamin and herbal program for your high blood pressure

Young individuals who are diagnosed with malignant hypertension need a further work-up. The work needs to done to exclude the possibility of a tumor on the adrenal gland that excretes epinephrine, also called adrenaline. The other condition is a narrowing of the aorta, which, if left untreated, can result in malignant hypertension and aortic tears. Depending on the location of this narrowing, the right-sided blood pressure will be higher than the left-sided blood pressure.

Q. My friend has been diagnosed with high blood pressure. She does not want to be placed on conventional blood pressure medications. She is starting to use acupuncture. Do you believe that acupuncture and Chinese herbs should be used in the treatment of lowering her blood pressure?

A. Traditional Chinese medicine is a well-established, researched method for treatment of a wide variety of diseases, including hypertension. Their method involves the use of Chinese herbs, acupuncture, massage, and energy medicine to lower blood pressure. In our office, we do use acupuncture, reiki, and Chinese herbs to reduce high blood pressure, as well as stress. Our acupuncturist focuses on bringing balance back to the liver and kidneys. Some Chinese practitioners have used bupleurum to disperse liver energy, thus lowering blood pressure.

Q. How long can a person survive with very low blood pressure? My mom is in the hospital and her top number was

50 and her bottom number was too low to read? How long can she survive?

A. Hypotension, or low blood pressure, is a common condition. There are many conditions that can cause low blood pressure. Patients with congestive heart failure on medications and aortic stenosis have low pressure readings. Also, patients with a dilated cardiomyopathy (dilation of the heart) have low blood pressures. Some individuals are asymptomatic with systolic (top) pressures at 90 and a diastolic (bottom) at 60. However, a systolic pressure reading of 50, as indicated above, carries a serious prognosis. A low blood pressure could be due to cardiovascular collapse caused by a multitude of reasons, including, but not limited to, a heart attack or overwhelming infection.

Conclusion

This book was written with the intention of providing the public with alternative solutions to managing heart disease, and I believe we have done that. As you can see, there are many approaches and techniques that can be employed, depending on individual needs and circumstances.

The opinions and suggestions mentioned in this book represent, of course, only one set of options, but they are based on years of experience with a wide-ranging patient profile base. We have done our best to give you the most useful, up-to-date information we have in the hopes that you might recognize your own needs and now have some of the solutions to meet those needs.

It is up to you, the patient, to be your own best activist. It is not only recommended, but it is necessary that each of you take an active role in managing your health and preventing illness. Ask questions, get involved, and investigate potential alternatives instead of giving in to standard protocols that may not ring true to your personal beliefs. If this book has opened your eyes to the potential that exists in alternative health care, then we authors have been a success. Knowledge is power; and now that you possess this knowledge, it is up to each of you to utilize it.

Live long and live well!

Glossary

Angioplasty—the mechanical treatment of an atherosclerotic plaque by the use of an inflated balloon that is introduced into the coronary artery via a tube passed to the heart from the groin

Aneurysm—dilation or rupture of an artery, which can occur anywhere in the arterial system

Angina—the medical term for chest pain; occurs when there is coronary artery blockage; less blood flow means less oxygen

Angiogram—a study of the heart performed by passing catheters into the heart arteries and injecting dye

Aorta—the body's largest artery

Arrhythmias—abnormal heart rhythms; can generate from the atria or the ventricles

Atherosclerosis—known as hardening of the arteries

Atria—the top two (left and right) chambers of the heart

Atrial Fibrillation—an abnormal, irregular rhythm of the heart originating from the top chambers of the heart; the rhythms can be fast or slow

Benign Prostatic Hypertrophy—enlargement of the prostate gland

Calcium Channel Blockers—a class of heart medications that are used to treat high blood pressure and abnormal heart rhythms

Cardiomyopathy—dilation of the heart with a loss of muscle function; there are several types of cardiomyopathy: obstructive, restrictive, and dilated

Carotid Endarterectomy—a surgical procedure to remove a blockage of the carotid arteries

Cerebrovascular accident—a term for stroke; can occur from a blockage of one of the cerebral arteries or from a ruptured cerebral aneurysm

Chelation—to chelate is a word derived from Greek meaning "grab onto" as a "crab does"; chelation binds to or grabs onto minerals and toxic metals and removes them from the body; the most common chelating agent is EDTA, used to treat lead toxicity for atherosclerosis

Chronic Obstructive Pulmonary Disease—also known as emphysema; weakening and unwanted elasticity of the lung's air sacs

Claudication—the interruption or tightening of blood flow to a region of the body resulting in pain

Congestive Heart Failure—a dilation of the heart; causes include heart-valve disease, coronary artery disease, and heart-muscle disease; medically managed with medications to prevent symptoms; surgically managed with a cardiac transplant if not contraindicated

Coronary Artery Disease—atherosclerosis of the blood supply of the heart; partial blockage or total blockage can occur

C-reactive protein (CRP)—a protein that, when elevated, indicates inflammation and possible infection; the cardiac CRP, or high-sensitivity CRP (hs-CRP) indicates inflammation of the coronary arteries and associated with increased atherosclerosis; normal levels are less than 0.5 mg/dL

Coumadin—trade name for warfarin; an anticoagulant

Defibrillator—a mechanical device implanted in an individual to administer a precise electrical shock when the individual is suffering from a dangerous abnormal heart rhythm

Diabetes—a multifaceted disease characterized by an abnormal blood sugar and insulin level; there are two classic types: Type I, insulin dependent, and Type II, adult onset and not insulin dependent

Electron Beam Computed Tomography (EBCT)—a scan to determine the extent of calcium blockage in each individual coronary artery

Echocardiogram—a sonogram (ultrasound) of the heart to view the valves of the heart as well as the muscle pumping function

Ejection Fraction—the pumping function of the heart; normal ejection fraction is 55 to 75%

Electrocardiogram—a study of the electrical tracings of the heart

Enhanced External Counterpulsation (EECP)—a treatment for coronary artery disease whereby pressurized cuffs are applied to the legs; this augments the blood flow to coronary arteries, eventually resulting in new, collateral circulation and thus bypassing blocked arteries. This is a-traumatic, noninvasive treatment administered for 35 days

Fibrinogen—a clotting factor; there is a correlation between elevated fibrinogen levels and coronary artery disease; the acceptable range for fibrinogen is less than 300 mg/dL

Glucose Tolerance Test—a sampling of blood every hour for glucose and insulin in response to the ingestion of a standardized amount of sugar; this is a sensitive screening test for diabetes, early diabetes, and insulin sensitivity

Heart palpitations—a common term for extra heartbeats; medically are called premature ventricular or premature atrial contractions

Hematuria—a medical term for blood in the urine

Homocysteine—an amino acid that at abnormal levels (greater than 15) predisposes one to premature vascular damage or atherosclerosis; it is converted from a good amino acid, methionine, when there is a deficiency in vitamins B_6, B_{12}, and folic acid

Hyperlipidemia—an elevation in the lipid profile, which includes total cholesterol, low-density lipoprotein (LDL), high-density lipoprotein (HDL), and triglycerides

Hypertension—the medical term for high blood pressure

Hypoglycemia—the medical term for a low blood sugar

Hypothyroidism—a medical term for an underactive thyroid; this is detected by such symptoms as hair loss, fatigue, weight gain, and low body temperatures; a blood test such as thyroid-stimulating hormone level, if too high, is a marker for hypothyroidism

Lipids—a broad class of compounds including fatty acids and cholesterol; in medicine, the term is used to refer to circulating lipid-containing particles, such as LDL, HDL, IDL, and VLDL

Lipoprotein(a)—a low-density lipoprotein; a gluelike substance; elevations are a risk factor for atherosclerosis; normal levels are less than 20; an independent risk factor for coronary artery disease; it is not diminished with the use of statin drugs

Longevity Risk Factors™—this is a term Dr. Fratellone coined to describe the other risk factors for atherosclerosis, independent of lipid levels; these risk factors include homocysteine, fibrinogen, lipoprotein(a), cardiac C-reactive protein, and iron levels

Myocardial Infarction—a medical term for heart attack; this is a complete occlusion of one the coronary arteries that supply blood to a wall of the heart

Nanobacterium sanguineum—a bacteria that has been found to excrete calcium; it can be associated with coronary artery calcification, kidney stones, prostate and breast calcifications, and atherosclerosis of other vascular structures

Peripheral Vascular Disease—atherosclerotic blockages and decreased blood flow in the arteries that supply the extremities of the body

Platelet—a circulating blood component that is involved in the clotting process

Plaque—the lesion of atherosclerosis

Plaquex®—this is the trade name for intravenous phosphatidylcholine, also known as *lecithin*

Renal System—the medical term for the kidneys

Silent Angina—the term *angina* by itself refers to decreased blood flow to the heart, resulting in decreased oxygen, and thus causing chest pain; silent angina is present in individuals who have blockage without symptoms; most commonly seen in diabetics

Statin—informal name for a class of drugs to reduce cholesterol by blocking the enzyme HMG-CoA reductase ; the most common prescribed drug is Lipitor®; the statin drugs deplete a vital nutrient for the body and the heart: CoQ_{10}

Stenosis—a narrowing of an artery usually caused by a plaque

Stent—a device placed in an artery to keep the artery open; stents can be placed in the coronary arteries.

Stress Test—a noninvasive test to determine if there is a coronary artery blockage; the exercise portion can be done on a bicycle or treadmill; during the test, the patient undergoes monitoring of blood pressure and pulse and a electrocardiogram is recorded; there are various types of stress tests: echo stress, thallium stress, and persantine thallium stress tests

Syndrome X—a syndrome characterized by insulin resistance, obesity, high triglycerides, and hypertension

Systolic Blood Pressure—the pressure the blood generates at the peak of heart contraction; this is the higher number, and is the top number in a reading

Tachycardia—a medical term referring to heart rates greater than 100 beats per minute; if the rhythm is normal and greater than 100, the term is *sinus tachycardia*; however, other rhythms can originate from other areas of heart and be greater than 100

Thrombosis—a medical term for a clot

Triglycerides—the medical term for the binding of three fatty acids to glycerol molecule; this is considered a risk factor for the development of coronary artery disease and diabetes

Valvular Heart Disease—a medical term collectively used for disorders of the valves; these can involve any of the four heart valves; the valves can either be regurgitant (leaky) or stenotic (tight)

Ventricle—the main pumping chambers of the heart; located at the bottom; there are two ventricles, one right and one left

Bibliography

Atha, Anthony: The Ultimate Herb Book. The Definitive Guide to growing and using over 200 Herbs. Collins and Brown. 2001.

Atkins, R.: Vita Nutrient Solution.

Bayer Voluntarily Withdraws Baycol. FDA Talk Papers: T01-34. August 8, 2001.

Blumenthal, M: Complete German Commission E Monographs. Therapeutic Guide to Herbal Medicines. 1998.

Colbert, D.: Walking in Divine Health. Siloam: Strang Publications. 1999.

Cranton, E.: Bypassing Bypass Surgery. Hampton Roads Publishing. 2001.

Deron, S.: C-Reactive Protein. Contemporary Books. 2004

Diamond, W. J., Cowden, W. L., and Goldberg, B.: Alternative Medicine Guide Cancer Diagnosis. Future Medicine Publishing. 1998.

Goldberg, B.: Alternative Medicine Guide to Heart Disease. Future Medicine Publishing. 1998.

Hoffman, D.: The Complete Illustrated Herbal. Barnes and Noble. 1999.

Jonas, W., and Levin, J. S.: Essentials of Complementary and Alternative Medicine. Lippincott, Williams and Wilkins. 1999.

Kaufmann, D. A.: The Fungus Link Volume 2. Media Trition. 2003.

Mahan, K., and Escott-Stump, S.: Krause's Food, Nutrition, and Diet Therapy. Saunders. 11th edition. 2000.

Mills, S., and Bone, K.: Principles and Practice of Phytotherapy, Churchill Livingston. 2000.

Murray, M. T.: The Healing Power of Herbs. Prima Publishing. 1995.

O'Neill, K., and Murray, B.: Power Plants. Woodland Publishing. 2002

Oz, M.: Healing from the Heart. Penguin Books. 1998.

PDR for Herbal Medicines: Medical Economic Publisher 2000.

Professional Guide to Conditions, Herbs, and Supplements. Integrative Medicine. 2000.

Ravnskov, U.: The Cholesterol Myths. New Trends Publishing. 2000.

Sinatra, S.: The Coenzyme Q10 Phenomenon. Keats Publishing 1998.

Skidmore-Roth, L.: Mosby's Handbook of Herbs and Natural Supplements. 2nd Edition. 2004.

Stockton S.: Beyond Amalgam. The Hidden Health Hazard Posed by Jawbone Cavitations. Power of One Publishing 1998.

Superko, R.: Before the Heart Attacks. 2003

Yannois, T.: The Heart Disease Breakthrough. The 10-Step Program That Can Save Your Life. John Wiley and Sons. 1999.

About the Fratellone Group for Integrative Cardiology and Medicine

The Fratellone Group for Integrative Cardiology and Medicine, located in mid-town Manhattan, was established in October, 2002, by Patrick Fratellone, MD. Prior to opening his own private practice, Dr. Fratellone was the chief of medicine and director of cardiology for the Atkins Center for Complementary Medicine under the late Robert C. Atkins, MD. The Fratellone Group is dedicated to serving patients committed to their own well-being. We also believe that the mind and body are connected and, thus, have an effect on the state of health.

Dr. Fratellone treats heart disease through the use of conventional testing as well as alternative therapies. This approach enables him to detect problems early and treat patients with an aggressive nutritional approach in order to prevent stroke and heart attack. In addition to heart disease, the Fratellone Group also treats a wide variety of other disorders, including diabetes, cancers, asthma, thyroid, arthritis, HIV/AIDS, hepatitis, autoimmune diseases, chronic fatigue, multiple sclerosis, and Alzheimer's and Parkinson's diseases.

The Fratellone Group is dedicated to

- Empowering patients to take a more active role in their health care, bringing traditional and alternative approaches to well-being

- Working as a team with other alternative and conventional practitioners, including nutritionists, physician assistants, and nurses

- Promoting and providing natural health services to the community

- Educating the public about natural medicine and encouraging an appreciation of our connection to all humanity and to nature

For information on becoming a patient of the Fratellone Group, please call our new patient number at 212-977-1539.

The Fratellone Group for Integrative Cardiology and Medicine
Patrick Fratellone, MD
Executive Medical Director
24 West 57th Street, Suite 701
New York, New York 10019
www.thefratellonegroup.com

About Longevity Nutritional Products and Services

To address the diverse and individual needs of Fratellone Group patients, as well as numerous others who follow Dr. Fratellone's medical and nutritional philosophies, Dr. Fratellone has authorized the development of numerous vita-nutrient products. These products are designed to provide the user with effective, user-friendly, targeted formulations that maximize the therapeutic benefits associated with specific vita-nutrients. Furthermore, these nutrients are continually updated to include the purest and highest-quality materials identified through research, to enhance the effectiveness of these products.

For more information on products available from Longevity Nutritionals, Inc., please call 1-800-543-7989 or visit their website, at www.longevitynutritionals.com.

Index

A
absorption rate 4
ACAM 48
acetylcholine 24
adaptogenic herb 19, 29, 30
alanine 30
alpha lipoic acid 15, 58
Alzheimer's disease 23, 24
amino acids 3, 18, 23, 28, 30, 51, 79, 88, 89
angina xiii, 37, 46, 47, 49, 95, 99
angioplasty xiv, 45, 47, 48, 59, 95
antibiotic 13, 81
antioxidant 11, 14, 21, 23, 24, 27, 37, 40, 49, 58
arrhythmias 9, 37, 39, 44, 56, 69, 70, 72, 73, 74, 75, 76, 78, 84, 95
arthritis 20, 21, 31, 40, 103
atherosclerosis 20, 39, 46, 48, 50, 55, 59, 95, 96, 98, 99
atrial fibrillation 36, 42, 69, 72, 73, 74, 75, 95
autoimmune 21, 103
Avena sativa 25

B
B12 vitamin 7, 9, 16
B6 vitamin 7
benign prostatic hyperplasia 30, 31
beta-blockers 7, 37, 41, 72, 73, 81, 84, 86
biotin 7, 32
black cohosh 36
bowel intolerance 12
bugleweed 37

C
calcium 7, 9, 10, 13, 48, 49, 50, 70, 72, 75, 76, 84, 89, 95, 97, 99
calcium channel blockers 7, 72, 95
carbohydrate 16, 64, 71
cardiomyopathy 44, 54, 55, 72, 78, 79, 82, 83, 91, 96
carnitine, L-carnitine 8, 20, 24, 25, 42, 45, 79, 81, 83, 84, 88, 89
cerebrovascular accident 96
cetyl myristoleate 21
chelation xv, 45, 48, 49, 56, 60, 75, 96
chlamydial species 47
cholesterol xiii, xiv, 10, 12, 13, 14, 17, 19, 20, 22, 23, 25, 26, 29, 31, 38, 40, 46, 48, 51, 52, 58, 62, 63, 64, 65, 98, 99, 102
chromium 12, 13, 17, 22, 58, 72, 88
chromium picolinate 17, 22
chronic obstructive pulmonary disease (COPD) 56
Coenzyme Q10 (CoQ10) 4, 82
congestive heart failure xiii, 36, 37, 44, 72, 78, 80, 81, 83, 84, 85, 91, 96
conjugated linoleic acid 23
contraindicated 7, 96
conventional medications 2, 7, 8, 23, 34, 37, 39, 56, 59, 72, 78, 81, 83, 87, 88
coral calcium 9

coronary artery disease xiii, 44, 45, 46, 47, 50, 51, 52, 54, 58, 62, 64, 66, 67, 69, 71, 79, 85, 86, 96, 97, 98, 100
Coumadin 6, 40, 58, 59, 61, 69, 73, 82, 96
C-reactive protein xiv, 11, 19, 25, 33, 40, 46, 55, 63, 74, 96, 98, 101
cruciferous vegetables 19, 61
cystic acne 13
cytomegalovirus 47

D

dandelion leaf 42
defibrillator 55, 56, 97
detoxification 26, 27
Diabetes type I 57
Diabetes type II 57
diet xv, 3, 4, 6, 10, 18, 19, 26, 31, 46, 56, 61, 62, 63, 64, 65, 66, 67, 76, 102
dihydrotestosterone 31

E

echinacea 36
echocardiogram 39, 48, 54, 70, 81, 89, 97
EDTA 48, 49, 50, 56, 60, 96
ejection fraction 48, 49, 51, 56, 79, 83, 97
electrocardiogram 39, 48, 54, 81, 97, 100
endarterectomy 60, 96
enhanced external counterpulsation (EECP) 79, 97
enzyme 14, 58, 78, 88, 99
epidemic 66
essential oils 9, 14, 20, 21, 25, 51, 52

F

fenugreek 58
fibrinogen xiv, 11, 12, 19, 31, 38, 47, 50, 51, 55, 63, 97, 98
flatulence 21
flax seed oils 11, 19

folic acid 7, 9, 10, 16, 20, 76, 98
foxglove 36, 37, 72

G

garlic 20, 38, 81
gelatin capsules 3
ginger 21, 40
Ginkgo biloba 14, 20, 24, 25, 30, 39, 52, 81
ginseng 19, 24, 28, 29, 30, 33
glucose 15, 16, 17, 22, 23, 57, 66, 73, 74, 97
glucose tolerance test 15, 16, 57, 66, 73, 74, 97
glutathione peroxidase 14
glycine 30
gymnema 58

H

hawthorn 9, 36, 37, 39, 41, 70, 80, 81, 86, 88, 89
HDL 46, 52, 63, 64, 65, 98
heart palpitations 18, 23, 97
heavy metal intoxication 24
Helicobacter pylori 47
hematuria 98
herbs xv, 2, 3, 6, 7, 8, 16, 19, 20, 21, 24, 25, 29, 30, 31, 32, 33, 35, 36, 37, 39, 40, 41, 42, 44, 45, 55, 56, 57, 58, 70, 72, 76, 77, 78, 79, 80, 81, 83, 84, 86, 87, 88, 89, 90, 101, 102
Herpes simplex 47
homocysteine xiv, 11, 19, 46, 50, 51, 55, 63, 98
horse chestnut 39
hyperlipidemia 44, 62, 63, 98
hypertension xiii, xiv, 30, 37, 41, 44, 59, 80, 84, 85, 86, 87, 89, 90, 98, 100
hypoallergenic 5
hypoglycemia 49, 57, 74, 98

hypoglycemic 14
hypothyroidism 23, 32, 33, 98

I
immune system dysfunction 7
impotence xiv, 30, 72
inflammation 21, 25, 31, 33, 34, 40, 46, 47, 50, 51, 56, 96
insomnia 18, 23, 36, 39, 42, 77
insulin levels 16, 57, 66, 74
intravenous 24, 45, 56, 76, 99
invasive xiv, xv, 45, 47, 56, 73

K
kelp 18

L
l-carnitine 8, 20, 24, 81, 88, 89
LDL xiii, 46, 51, 62, 63, 64, 65, 66, 98
lead intoxication 48
libido 24, 30, 33
lily of the valley 37, 42, 72
linden flowers 41
lipoprotein(a) xiv, 11, 19, 50, 51, 55, 63, 65, 98
Longevity Risk Factors xiv, 11, 19, 38, 40, 48, 50, 63, 89, 98
l-taurine 20, 81, 84, 88, 89
lycopene 30

M
macronutrients 6
macular degeneration 7
magnesium 9, 20, 25, 42, 56, 70, 72, 74, 76, 80, 81, 84, 86, 88, 89
metabolic syndromes 66
milk thistle 26
minerals xi, xv, 2, 3, 4, 5, 6, 9, 10, 22, 30, 32, 34, 49, 57, 72, 80, 84, 96

mistletoe 39
motherwort 37, 70, 72, 77
MSM 21, 57
mycoplasmal species 47
myocardial infarction 46, 99
myristoleic acid 21

N
N-acetyl-cysteine 27
NADH 24
Nanobacterium sanguineum 47, 99
neti pot 22
neuropathy 15
niacin 7, 25, 51, 63, 64, 65, 67, 68
night blooming cactus 37, 70, 72
noninvasive 45, 50, 79, 97, 100
nutrients 1, 2, 3, 4, 5, 6, 11, 14, 15, 22, 23, 24, 25, 26, 29, 31, 32, 47, 88, 105

O
obesity xiii, 53, 62, 66, 100
omega-3 9, 11, 17, 31, 38, 47, 58, 90
osteoarthritis 14, 20
osteoporosis 9, 10, 13, 53

P
pantothenic acid 7, 32
Parkinson's disease 13, 24, 42, 83, 103
passion flower 41, 42, 77
PDR 7, 34, 102
periodontal infections 47
phenylalanine 18, 23
phosphatidylcholine 49, 56, 99
plaque 38, 45, 46, 47, 48, 49, 50, 58, 95, 99
plaque rupture 46
Plaquex xv, 49, 50, 56, 75, 99
platelet 14, 38, 40, 47, 99
prostate gland 25, 30, 31, 95

R

refined carbohydrates 6, 17, 18, 62, 66, 74
regurgitant 48, 70, 78, 100
renal system 41, 99
rheumatoid arthritis 21
rhodiola root 30
riboflavin 7

S

sarsaparilla 24, 33
saturated fats 16, 63
saw palmetto 30, 31, 32
scotch broom 37, 72
selenium 9, 14, 30
senile plaques 23
Siberian ginseng 24, 33
silent angina 46, 99
sinusitis 20, 21, 22
skullcap 39, 77
soy 19
St. John's wort 36, 77
stabilized glucose levels 13, 17, 23
statin drug xiv, 14, 51, 63, 64, 98, 99
stenosis 54, 55, 59, 60, 91, 99
stenotic 48, 70, 78, 100
stent 39, 45, 47, 48, 60, 99
stress test 48, 56, 71, 75, 89, 100
stroke xiii, 20, 38, 41, 45, 46, 47, 51, 59, 60, 69, 86, 96, 103

T

tachycardia 30, 37, 42, 56, 73, 75, 100
testosterone 24, 31
thiamin 7, 84
thrombosis 100
thyroid 14, 18, 19, 23, 32, 33, 69, 71, 77, 98, 103
tinctures 41
trace minerals 9, 49
turmeric 21, 40
tyrosine 18, 23

V

valerian 36, 39, 76
valvular heart disease 44, 78, 79, 83, 84, 85, 100
vitamin C 7, 9, 10, 12, 20, 27, 40, 49, 51, 57, 72, 88
vitamin E 6, 7, 9, 14, 24, 25, 30, 51, 52, 88
vitamin toxicity 5
vitamins xi, xv, 2, 3, 4, 5, 6, 7, 8, 9, 11, 12, 16, 18, 19, 22, 23, 24, 25, 26, 30, 32, 34, 51, 55, 56, 61, 63, 65, 66, 67, 70, 73, 76, 78, 81, 83, 84, 86, 87, 88, 89, 98
vita-nutrients 1, 2, 88, 105

W

water soluble 19

Y

yohimbine 30

0-595-66660-4